The Art of Peace and Relaxation *Workbook*

SEVENTH EDITION

Brian Luke Seaward, PhD
Paramount Wellness Institute
Boulder, Colorado

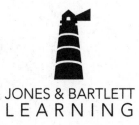

JONES & BARTLETT
LEARNING

World Headquarters
Jones & Bartlett Learning
5 Wall Street
Burlington, MA 01803
978-443-5000
info@jblearning.com
www.jblearning.com

Jones & Bartlett Learning Canada
6339 Ormindale Way
Mississauga, Ontario L5V 1J2
Canada

Jones & Bartlett Learning International
Barb House, Barb Mews
London W6 7PA
United Kingdom

Jones & Bartlett Learning books and products are available through most bookstores and online booksellers. To contact Jones & Bartlett Learning directly, call 800-832-0034, fax 978-443-8000, or visit our website, www.jblearning.com.

Substantial discounts on bulk quantities of Jones & Bartlett Learning publications are available to corporations, professional associations, and other qualified organizations. For details and specific discount information, contact the special sales department at Jones & Bartlett Learning via the above contact information or send an email to specialsales@jblearning.com.

Production Credits
Senior Acquisitions Editor: Shoshanna Goldberg
Editorial Assistant: Prima Bartlett
Production Manager: Julie Champagne Bolduc
Production Editor: Jessica Steele Newfell
Production Assistant: Sean Coombs
Associate Marketing Manager: Jody Sullivan
V.P., Manufacturing and Inventory Control: Therese Connell
Composition: Cenveo Publisher Services
Cover Design: Kate Ternullo
Photo Researcher: Sarah Cebulski
Cover Image: © Brian Luke Seaward
Printing and Binding: Courier Kendallville
Cover Printing: Courier Kendallville

Photo Credits: **Page 74** © John Lock/ShutterStock, Inc.; **pages 118, 172, 173, 205, 208** © Sergio Hayashi/ ShutterStock, Inc.

Unless otherwise indicated, all photographs and illustrations are under copyright of Jones & Bartlett Learning, or have been provided by the author.

ISBN: 978-1-4496-3438-4

6048
Printed in the United States of America
15 14 13 12 11   10 9 8 7 6 5 4 3 2 1

Contents

Contents

Contents

Contents

To Know and Not to Do
Is Not to Know

Stress is the equal-opportunity destroyer. It affects everyone: rich and poor, young and old, male and female. You can learn all the concepts of stress management (and many people do), but actually using the techniques and putting the skills to practice is another story. Sadly, good stress management is common sense, but common sense is not too common when people are continually stressed out in a fast-paced, 24/7 society. Instead they claim victimization ("poor, poor pitiful me") and proceed to perpetuate the stress-prone thoughts and behaviors that, in turn, attract even more stress.

There is a saying relevant to this situation: "To know and not to do is not to know." Simply stated, you can learn the best coping skills and the best relaxation techniques in the world, but if you don't practice them, what good are they? They're wasted knowledge.

This workbook contains more than 140 exercises in the form of surveys, questionnaires, inventories, and journal entries, all for the purpose of engaging you to make some or all of these skills part of your daily routine so that you can achieve balance and stop feeling like a victim. Although it is best to read the corresponding chapter in the text, *Managing Stress*, before you begin the workbook exercises, for most exercises it isn't necessary. Moreover, by doing these exercises you will find they become a great study guide for the textbook. By combining effective coping skills (mind) and effective relaxation techniques (body), the goal is frequent and quality periods of homeostasis. First and foremost, stress management is experiential. You learn by doing—there is no other way! This is the purpose of all of these exercises. You may find that different exercises seem to be similar in content. The reason is simple: People have different learning styles and may respond to one exercise more than another until a critical mass is formed and the lightbulb finally goes off over the head. In this case, the lightbulb is achieving integration: balance and harmony of mind, body, spirit, and emotions.

It may be a cliché (remember that clichés are based on simple truths), but you only get out of this workbook what you put into it. Please take time with each exercise. Be honest with yourself. Answer the questions as you are, not how you want to be or wish you were. Time (as expressed through discipline) and honesty are two of the most important criteria for effectively changing your behavior so that, indeed, you can live a healthier, happier life.

The Nature of Stress

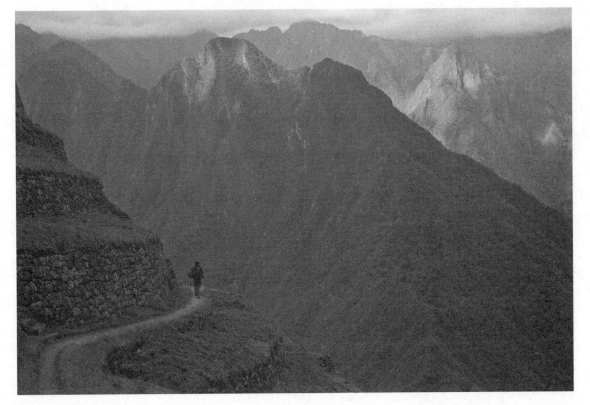

The Nature of Stress

EXERCISE **1.1**

Inventory: Are You Stressed?

Although there is no definitive survey composed of twenty to forty questions to determine whether you are stressed or burnt out, or exactly how stressed you really are, questionnaires do help increase awareness that, indeed, there may be a problem in one or more areas of your life. The following is an example of a simple stress inventory to help you determine the level of stress in your life. Read each statement and then circle either the word Agree or Disagree. Then count the number of "Agree" answers you've circled (scoring one point per answer) and use the stress level key to determine your personal stress level.

Statement	*Agree*	*Disagree*
1. I have a hard time falling asleep at night.	Agree	Disagree
2. I tend to suffer from tension and/or migraine headaches.	Agree	Disagree
3. I find myself thinking about finances and making ends meet.	Agree	Disagree
4. I wish I could find more to laugh and smile about each day.	Agree	Disagree
5. More often than not, I skip breakfast or lunch to get things done.	Agree	Disagree
6. If I could change my job situation, I would.	Agree	Disagree
7. I wish I had more personal time for leisure pursuits.	Agree	Disagree
8. I have lost a good friend or family member recently.	Agree	Disagree
9. I am unhappy in my relationship or am recently divorced.	Agree	Disagree
10. I haven't had a quality vacation in a long time.	Agree	Disagree
11. I wish that my life had a clear meaning and purpose.	Agree	Disagree
12. I tend to eat more than three meals a week outside the home.	Agree	Disagree
13. I tend to suffer from chronic pain.	Agree	Disagree
14. I don't have a strong group of friends to whom I can turn.	Agree	Disagree
15. I don't exercise regularly (more than three times per week).	Agree	Disagree
16. I am on prescribed medication for depression.	Agree	Disagree
17. My sex life is not very satisfying.	Agree	Disagree

Statement	Agree	Disagree
18. My family relationships are less than desirable.	Agree	(Disagree)
19. Overall, my self-esteem can be rather low.	(Agree)	Disagree
20. I spend no time each day dedicated to meditation or centering.	(Agree)	Disagree

Stress Level Key

Less than 5 points	You have a low level of stress and maintain good coping skills.
More than 5 points	You have a moderate level of personal stress.
More than 10 points	You have a high level of personal stress.
More than 15 points	You have an exceptionally high level of stress.

* (12) high level of personal stress

EXERCISE **1.2**

My Health Philosophy

Life is a kaleidoscope of the infinite variety. No two things
are the same. Everyone's life is individual.
Paramahansa Yogananda

We all have philosophies. Philosophies are nothing more than our opinions, dressed up with an introduction and conclusion—a way to present to someone, even ourselves, what we really think about some topic or ideal. We have philosophies on everything—the types of music we like and listen to, the state of world affairs, and even the foods we eat at restaurants.

Now it's time to examine your philosophy about your health. Based on what you already know, and perhaps have been taught or exposed to, define as best you can what the words *health* and *wellness* mean to you. After having done this, ask yourself why health is so important and write a few lines about this.

Given the premise that every issue is a health issue, identify some seemingly nonhealth issues such as the global economy, deforestation, or TV programming. See if you can discover the connection between these issues and your state of well-being. How is your state of health influenced by stress? Finally, where do you see yourself 25 years from now? If you were to continue your current lifestyle for the next three to four decades, how do you see yourself at that point in the future? Your health philosophy guides your state of health. What is your health philosophy? What has influenced your philosophy up to now (e.g., parents, teachers, friends, books)? Be specific. Take some time to write it down here now. If you need additional space to write, use the extra pages provided at the back of this book.

My Health Philosophy

_____

_____

_____

_____

_____

_____

_____

_____

EXERCISE **1.3**

Self-Assessment: Poor Sleep Habits Questionnaire

Please take a moment to answer these questions based on your typical behavior. If you feel your sleep quality is compromised, consider that one or more of these factors may contribute to patterns of insomnia by affecting your physiology, circadian rhythms, or emotional thought processing. Although there is no key to determine your degree of insomnia, each question is based on specific factors associated with either a good night's sleep or the lack of it. Use each question to help you fine-tune your "sleep hygiene."

1. Do you go to bed at about the same time every night?   Yes   No

2. Does it take you more than 30 minutes to fall asleep once in bed?   Yes   No

3. Do you wake up at about the same time every day?   Yes   No

4. Do you drink coffee, tea, or caffeinated soda after 6 P.M.?   Yes   No

5. Do you watch television from your bed?   Yes   No

6. Do you perform cardiovascular exercise three to five times per week?   Yes   No

7. Do you use your bed as your office (e.g., homework, balancing checkbook, writing letters, etc.)?   Yes   No

8. Do you take a hot shower or bath before you go to sleep?   Yes   No

9. Do you have one or more drinks of alcohol before bedtime?   Yes   No

10. Are you engaged in intense mental activity before bed (e.g., term papers, exams, projects, reports, finances, taxes)?   Yes   No

11. Is your bedroom typically warm or even hot before you go to bed?   Yes   No

12. Does your sleep partner snore or become restless in the night?   Yes   No

13. Is the size and comfort level of your bed satisfactory?   Yes   No

14. Do you suffer from chronic pain while lying down?   Yes   No

15. Is your sleep environment compromised by noise, light, or pets?   Yes   No

16. Do you frequently take naps during the course of a day?   Yes   No

17. Do you take medications (e.g., decongestants, steroids, antihypertensives, asthma medications, or medications for depression)?   Yes   No

18. Do you tend to suffer from depression?   Yes   No

19. Do you eat a large, heavy meal right before you go to bed?   Yes   No

20. Do you use a cell phone regularly, particularly in the evening?   Yes   No

© 2012 Jones & Bartlett Learning, LLC

EXERCISE **1.4**

A Good Night's Sleep

Sleep is one of the basic human drives. Most health books don't talk much about it, despite the fact that you spend over one-third of your life in that state. The fact is that we tend to take the behavior of sleep for granted, unless, of course, we feel we don't get enough of it. We are told that the average person sleeps six to eight hours a night, with an occasional nap here and there. Truth be told, over half of Americans get much less than this. Eight hours may be recommended, but it is not the norm. A poor night's sleep cascades into a poor waking day. Over time, the results will ultimately affect all aspects of health.

Whatever your sleep patterns were before you started college, chances are that they have changed dramatically since then. By and large, the freedom connected with college life tends to throw off sleep patterns. Instead of hitting the hay around 10 P.M. or 11 P.M., you might not lay your head on the pillow until 1 A.M. or 2 A.M. On weekends you may go to bed at sunrise, rather than waking up to see it. And let us not forget the all-nighters that tend to become habit forming during midterm and final exams.

Since the 1950s, scientists have been studying sleeping behaviors and sleeping patterns in earnest. With over forty years of data collection, you'd think they would have some solid answers; the truth is, no one really knows why we sleep. There are all kinds of theories about the need to have rest, but to date there seems to be a lack of evidence as to what actually goes on during the night hours. Interestingly enough, we *do* know what happens when we don't get enough sleep. Memory and motor coordination fade rapidly, and performance, in all aspects, is greatly compromised—as many a college student will attest to when pulling a series of all-nighters.

Describe your sleeping patterns. Are your sleep habits regular? Do you go to bed and get up about the same time every day? How have your sleeping patterns changed since you entered college? Do you make a habit of pulling all-nighters? Do you have problems sleeping at night? Do you have a hard time getting up in the morning? What are some of the patterns you see with your sleep?

_____

_____

_____

_____

_____

_____

_____

_____

_____

_____

_____

_____

_____

_____

_____

_____

_____

_____

_____

_____

_____

_____

_____

_____

EXERCISE **1.5**

Personal Stress Inventory: Top Ten Stressors

It's time to take a personal inventory of your current stressors—those issues, concerns, situations, or challenges that trigger the fight-or-flight response in your body. The first step to resolving any problem is learning to identify exactly what the problem is. Take a moment to list the top ten issues that you are facing at the present moment. Then place check marks in the columns to signify whether this stressor directly affects one or more aspects of your health (mind, body, spirit, emotions). Take note of how many of your stressors affect more than one aspect. Then, next to each stressor, chronicle how long it has been a problem. Finally, check whether this stressor is one that elicits some level of anger, fear, or both.

Stressor	Mental	Emotional	Spiritual	Physical	Duration of Problem
1.					
2.					
3.					
4.					
5.					
6.					
7.					
8.					
9.					
10.					

EXERCISE **1.6**

The Wellness Paradigm Revisited

Ageless wisdom tells us that the whole is greater than the sum of the parts and that all parts must be looked at equally as part of the whole. In terms of health and wellness, the whole is made up of four components: mind, body, spirit, and emotions. Additionally, ageless wisdom suggests that holistic wellness is composed of the integration, balance, and harmony of these four components—that each aspect of our being is so connected to the other three that no separations exist. Looking at one component—say, our physical health—merits paying attention to the other three because of the dynamic interconnectedness of the mind, body, spirit, and emotions. What might seem like common sense has not always been so well accepted in American culture. For over three hundred years, the Western mind has focused on the physical aspects of health, leaving the other three components in the shadows. Beginning in the early 1960s, the mental, emotional, and spiritual components of health were looked at with somewhat distant interest; only in the past decade has the interconnection of mind, body, and spirit gained respect (and popularity) in Western science.

It has been said recently that every issue is a health issue, meaning that issues such as economic downswings, political instability, rainforest depletion, and moral bankruptcy all ultimately affect our health. To recognize our own health status, we must remind ourselves that we are more than just our physical bodies. We must come to appreciate the true integration, balance, and harmony of mind, body, spirit, and emotions.

Here are some questions to ponder as you explore your own health philosophy, values, and beliefs. If you need additional space to write, use the extra pages provided at the back of the book.

1. Given the dynamics of the wellness paradigm, how does it compare with the common notion that health is the absence of disease?

2. What is your definition of wellness? Do you believe that the whole is greater than the sum of the parts? Can you think of an example in music, politics, or the arts that demonstrates this ageless wisdom?

3. What do you think it means to be an integrated person, to enjoy balance and harmony among your mental, emotional, physical, and spiritual aspects? Do you feel this within yourself? If not, why not? Can you identify which aspect(s) you feel are not in balance?

_____

_____

_____

_____

_____

EXERCISE **1.7**

The Circle: The Universal Symbol of Wholeness

The circle is a universal symbol of wholeness, as expressed in the American Indian medicine wheel, the Tibetan mandala, and many other symbols recognized worldwide. Typically these symbols depict four aspects, such as spring, summer, winter, and fall; mind, body, spirit, and emotions; or north, south, east, and west. This exercises invites you to increase your awareness of the power of this symbol.

1. List ten objects, found in nature, that symbolize wholeness (e.g., full moon, sun).

    1. _____
    2. _____
    3. _____
    4. _____
    5. _____
    6. _____
    7. _____
    8. _____
    9. _____
    10. _____

2. List ten objects or designs that are used in the American culture (or world culture) to convey a sense of wholeness to the unconscious mind (e.g., Starbucks logo, dinner plates, Christmas wreaths, the peace symbol).

    1. _____
    2. _____
    3. _____
    4. _____
    5. _____

6. _____

7. _____

8. _____

9. _____

10. _____

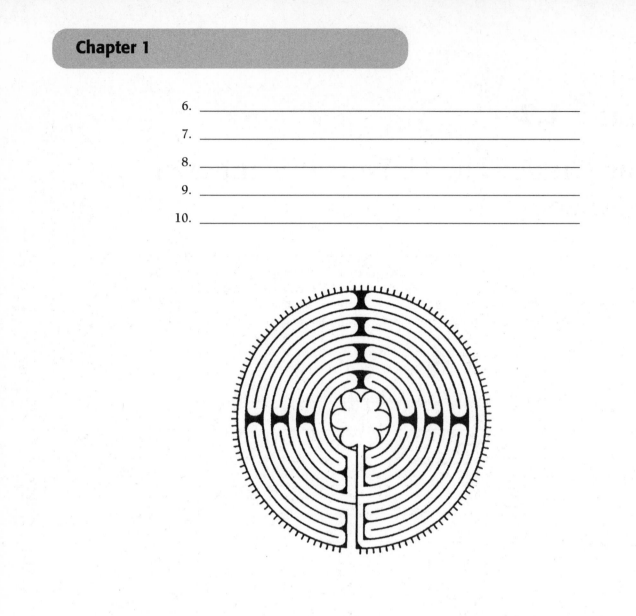

EXERCISE **1.8**

Daily Stressors Survey for College Students

It's a safe bet that you will hear the expression "real world" more than once while attending college—the real world being the noncollege world of long hours, hard work, and umpteen responsibilities. Years ago, the college experience was considered a luxury of the wealthy. For many rich kids, going to college was like taking a four-year vacation during which worldly responsibilities could be postponed, with the promise of a great job waiting after graduation. Times have changed since those Ivy League days of long ago. Going to college may not be the same thing as working on Wall Street or the emergency room of a local hospital, but college constitutes its own real world nonetheless. Being a college student comes with its own list of stressors, big and small. The following worksheet invites you to rank these typical daily student stressors (from 1 being low stress to 5 being high stress). In doing so, you take the first step in recognizing what issues need to be addressed in your current life situation.

Part I: How do these typical college student stressors rank in your life?

		LOW				HIGH
1.	Coping with roommates, living conditions	1	2	3	4	5
2.	Balancing schoolwork with job hours	1	2	3	4	5
3.	Making ends meet financially	1	2	3	4	5
4.	Academic load (credits, exams, papers)	1	2	3	4	5
5.	Social needs (friends, family, etc.)	1	2	3	4	5
6.	Health status, health issues	1	2	3	4	5
7.	Food, body image, and weight issues	1	2	3	4	5
8.	Transportation (car, traffic, gas, tickets)	1	2	3	4	5
9.	Parental issues, child care issues, etc.	1	2	3	4	5
10.	Girlfriend, boyfriend issues	1	2	3	4	5
11.	Technology problems (Facebook updates, text messages, RAM, etc.)	1	2	3	4	5
12.	Purpose-in-life issues	1	2	3	4	5

Part II: Please list any and all additional daily or weekly stressors and rank these as well.

		LOW				HIGH
1.	_____	1	2	3	4	5
2.	_____	1	2	3	4	5
3.	_____	1	2	3	4	5

		LOW				HIGH
4.	_____	1	2	3	4	5
5.	_____	1	2	3	4	5
6.	_____	1	2	3	4	5
7.	_____	1	2	3	4	5
8.	_____	1	2	3	4	5
9.	_____	1	2	3	4	5
10.	_____	1	2	3	4	5

Part III: Additional comments you wish to make:

_____

_____

_____

_____

_____

_____

_____

_____

_____

_____

_____

_____

_____

_____

_____

_____

_____

EXERCISE **1.9**

Stimulation Overload

In the early years of our lives, we crave sensory stimulation: loud music, fast-moving video games, movies, food—the list is nearly endless. All of this stimulation increases our threshold for excitement, and we seek more and more to reach this threshold of excitement. This sensory stimulation falls under the category of "good stress," that which motivates us and makes us happy. At some point, however, too much of a good thing can become bad. Too much sensory stimulation can become sensory overload, which then leads to burnout. *Burnout* is another word for bad stress. This exercise invites you to take an honest look at those things that you would consider good stress and how you manage them to maintain an optimal level of health and performance.

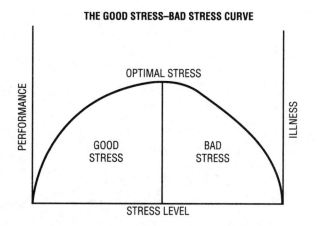

THE GOOD STRESS–BAD STRESS CURVE

1. What things do you crave for sensory stimulation? Make a list.

   _____

   _____

   _____

2. How do you know when you have had too much sensory stimulation (stimulation overload)? What are the signs or symptoms of personal burnout?

   _____

   _____

   _____

3. How has your threshold of excitement changed over the years? (If you are younger than 20, consider how your threshold differs from that of your parents and grandparents.)

_____

_____

_____

4. Do you see an association between too much sensory stimulation and your health status (good or bad)? Please explain.

_____

_____

_____

The Sociology of Stress

EXERCISE **2.1**

Are You a Product of Your Culture?

The following questions are based on various behaviors observed in individuals in society. Please answer each question as you really behave, not how you would like to be, by circling Yes or No as appropriate.

1.	I keep my cell phone on throughout the day so I won't miss any calls or texts.	**Yes**	No
2.	I use my Facebook account more often than my email account.	Yes	**No**
3.	I tend to leave the water running while brushing my teeth.	**Yes**	No
4.	I eat more than one prepared meal out of the house each day.	**Yes**	No
5.	During the day, I constantly check emails and text messages as they come in.	**Yes**	No
6.	I drive rather than take mass transit to and from work/college regularly.	**Yes**	No
7.	I typically take my laptop, BlackBerry, etc., on vacation with me.	Yes	**No**
8.	I have been known to flush unused medications down the toilet.	Yes	**No**
9.	I get more of my news from Comedy Central (e.g., *The Daily Show, The Colbert Report*) than newspapers, National Public Radio, TV news, or Internet portals.	Yes	**No**
10.	I spend less than one hour outside each day in a natural setting.	**Yes**	No
11.	I regularly interact (leave comments) on Web sites I visit.	Yes	**No**
12.	I find that I rely more and more on the Internet for information (e.g., MapQuest, Google) and less on memory retention.	Yes	**No**
13.	More often than not, I digitally record my favorite TV shows and watch them at a time of my preference.	**Yes**	No
14.	I recycle all cans, bottles, newspapers, and so forth.	**Yes**	No
15.	I start to feel antsy if I cannot check my email, text messages, and Facebook accounts each hour or more often.	Yes	**No**
16.	I spend more time inside playing video games or on the Internet than time spent outside in nature each day.	**Yes**	No
17.	I check my emails, tweets, Facebook updates, and so forth within 10 minutes of waking up each morning.	Yes	**No**

18. I have one or more tattoos as a means of self-expression.   Yes   No

19. I own more than one cell phone and often use them both at the same time (e.g., for phone calls, apps, Google).   Yes   No

20. I make more than one purchase online each week.   Yes   No

21. I dread answering the onslaught of emails each day.   Yes   No

22. I get a bit of a rush or excitement when my cell phone rings.   Yes   No

23. I text message my friends and parents more than I call them by phone.   Yes   No

24. I watch more movies via the Internet or Netflix than in a movie theater.   Yes   No

25. I make an effort to buy organic produce each week.   Yes   No

26. I have more than 50 Web sites bookmarked on my computer.   Yes   No

27. I have more than 250 friends on Facebook.   Yes   No

28. I purchase plastic water bottles rather than use a stainless steel one.   Yes   No

29. I have more than 25 apps on my smartphone.   Yes   No

30. I watch at least one YouTube video per day.   Yes   No

31. The majority of my purchases are via credit card or debit card, not cash.   Yes   No

32. I post an update to Facebook at least once a day.   Yes   No

33. I belong to more than one social networking Web site.   Yes   No

34. I prefer to read books on a Kindle or an iPad rather than printed books.   Yes   No

Results: The purpose of these questions is to increase your awareness of the impact the current culture has on your behavior. There is no definitive answer or "score" regarding the impact of cultural influences. We participate in cultural practices primarily as a means of being accepted. Most people are completely unaware of the influence that society has on them, unless they purposely act differently than cultural norms suggest.

EXERCISE **2.2**

The Age of Incivility

Always = 5   Often = 4   Sometimes = 3   Seldom = 2   Rarely = 1   Never = 0

1. I hold the door open for people when walking in or out of a store or building.   ____

2. If I use my cell phone in public, I find a quiet place away from people to talk.   ____

3. I make a habit of smiling at others, including store clerks, postal workers, and restaurant servers.   ____

4. I only use the express checkout lane in the grocery store when I have the suggested number of items, even when I'm in a hurry.   ____

5. When driving, I allow other drivers to cut in front of me.   ____

6. If I am at the movies with a friend, I will suspend all conversations during the film.   ____

7. While on the phone, I give my full attention to the call and don't multitask by checking emails or doing other things.   ____

8. I let people finish speaking before I say something or comment.   ____

9. I say the words *please* and *thank you* when requesting something.   ____

10. I don't use my cell phone while driving.   ____

11. I will pull a dollar out of my wallet or purse for a homeless person.   ____

12. If I receive a second call while talking on the phone, I will ignore the incoming call.   ____

13. When listening to my iPod while walking, jogging, or downhill skiing, I acknowledge the presence of others with a smile, nod, or comment.   ____

14. When others express political or religious beliefs that are different from mine, I shift the conversation to a different topic.   ____

15. I tend to censor the use of swear words in public.   ____

Key: There are no set standards for degrees of civility. Either you are or you are not! This survey is an awareness tool to examine your own behavior. If you score less than 30 points, you might consider changing your behavior, because most likely people see you as lacking in civility.

EXERCISE **2.3**

The Environmental Disconnect

How tuned in to the environment are you? Let's find out. Take this quick True/False quiz.

1. The majority of the ocean's coral reefs are dying due to agricultural runoff, poor fishing practices, and the formaldehyde used to capture tropical fish. True False

2. Over 60 percent of the food in your local grocery store is genetically modified. True False

3. About one-half of the world's population does not have drinkable water in their houses. True False

4. The acidity of the world's oceans is increasing at an alarming rate. True False

5. Wild salmon contain much less polychlorinated biphenyls (PCBs) than do those raised in fisheries. True False

6. The mercury found in coldwater fish comes from coal-burning plants used to make electricity for everyday use. True False

7. Hormones and antibiotics dumped into toilets are not filtered out in water treatment plants. True False

8. Experts predict that the ocean's natural fisheries will collapse in your lifetime. True False

9. It takes over 2,500 gallons of water to produce one hamburger. True False

10. On average, there are over 16 million new cars on the road every year. True False

11. Ethanol fuel still requires petrochemicals (oil) for its production (fertilizers, etc.). True False

12. Farm-raised salmon must take beta-carotene pellets so that the fish's flesh is pink/orange. True False

13. City light pollution is thought to be a contributing factor to the increase in insomnia across America. True False

14. The majority of food in your local grocery story has been transported over 1,500 miles to rest on those store shelves before being purchased. True False

15. Droughts in the Amazon rainforest contribute to global warming. True False

The answer for all of these questions is *true*. But don't get too stressed out. Being aware of each problem is half of the solution. Knowledge is power. Environmental disconnect is based largely on ignorance and apathy. Although some people choose to stick their heads in the sand, others are taking an active role toward living a sustainable life by changing their behaviors to become in sync with the environment. Although one person's life may seem insignificant to the big picture, nothing could be further from the truth. What can you do? Plenty!

List ten things that you do (or can start doing) to live a more sustainable lifestyle and reconnect with the biosphere on which we live—planet Earth.

1. _____
   _____
2. _____
   _____
3. _____
   _____
4. _____
   _____
5. _____
   _____
6. _____
   _____
7. _____
   _____
8. _____
   _____
9. _____
   _____
10. _____
   _____

EXERCISE **2.4**

It's All About Me: The Age of Narcissism

Enough about me. What do you think about me?
Bette Midler

Consider these facts: Today anyone can publish their own book, cut their own song, enter a photo contest, post their own blog, or make their own movie and gain world-wide attention, if not millions of fans, via YouTube. Reality shows are the rage on TV, from *Jersey Shore* to *Home Improvements*. Anyone can become a celebrity, specifically a "laptop celebrity." Experts who keep their fingers on the pulse of humanity are growing increasingly concerned. The "Me" generation has now expanded over several decades to include several generations. The self-absorbed, all-about-me, narcissistic, 15-minutes-of-fame culture is nothing more than the ego run amok.

The problems with unbridled egos (multiplied by 7 billion people) cannot be understated. If everyone is looking out only for themselves, then many people—and perhaps cultures, if not the world—will suffer. The American Psychiatric Association decided to delete narcissism disorder from its upcoming edition of the *Diagnostic and Statistical Manual of Mental Disorders* (DSM-5) in 2013, suggesting that this behavior is too common now to be recognized as a disorder.

Granted, you have to have some interest in yourself. After all, that's what self-esteem is all about. Balance is the key. At what point is the line crossed? That is the million-dollar question. The opposite of narcissism is altruism: doing something for others without any expectation of reciprocation—in essence, a random act of kindness.

1. Have you noticed that, in general, people are self-absorbed, perhaps even clueless about others who are eclipsed by their own stature? Are such people in denial about their inflated egos?

   _____

   _____

   _____

   _____

2. Have you been accused of being narcissistic, or simply full of yourself? Please explain.

   _____

   _____

   _____

   _____

3. How would you best describe your "presence" in the world? Do you have a Web site? A blog? Multiple YouTube video postings? Songs posted on Myspace.com? Books on Amazon? How many Facebook updates do you post per day? How many minutes have you used up from your allotment of 15 minutes of fame (or have you gone over this limit)?

_____

_____

_____

_____

4. Why do you suppose people are over the top regarding being self-righteous or simply fascinated with themselves? Is it a need for approval? Is it a need for acceptance? Is it a question of insecurity? What is your take on this new normal of the "Me" generation?

_____

_____

_____

_____

5. If indeed altruism is the polar opposite of narcissism, what actions do you take on a regular basis to seek balance? What do you do to domesticate your ego?

_____

_____

_____

_____

EXERCISE **2.5**

The Hidden Cost of "Convenience"

Technology has made some aspects of life very convenient. If you get lost driving, simply download an app to find your way. Want to tell someone you're going to be late for dinner? Text them. Afraid you might miss a special on television? TiVo it! Hungry? Grab some fast food at a convenience store. Hate your job? Send an email saying you quit. In a day and age where almost everything is "accessible," life, or many aspects of it, has become extremely convenient. Are the short-term gains worth the long-term risks, however? Is what is convenient to you uncivil to someone else? As with almost anything, there are drawbacks or hidden costs.

This workbook exercise invites you to take a hard look at the hidden costs of convenience, whether that is technology or any other aspects of society that might just come back and bite you in the butt. What are the social implications of the convenience factor? Before you write down any thoughts, think of times when what you thought may have been convenient for you turned out not to be. Then write a reaction paper regarding the hidden costs of convenience.

The Physiology of Stress

EXERCISE **3.1**

Stress Physiology Review

First, read Chapter 3 in *Managing Stress*. Given the nature of the content (lots of left-brain facts), you might want to reread it before starting this exercise. One reason why experts in mind-body medicine think it's a good idea to understand the physiology of stress is that this knowledge helps with various relaxation skills, including mental imagery, autogenic training, and biofeedback. Having this knowledge of how your body's physiology works during times of stress augments your ability to promote a deeper sense of relaxation and healing. In this case, knowledge is power.

This hormone is released from the hypothalamus:

1. _____

This hormone is released from the pituitary:

1. _____

This hormone is released from the thyroid:

1. _____

These hormones and catecholamines are released from the adrenal gland:

1. _____

2. _____

3. _____

4. _____

These catecholamines are released from the neural endings:

1. _____

2. _____

This hormone is associated with mood; a decrease is associated with depression:

1. _____

This hormone is associated with a good night's sleep:

1. _____

This hormone is associated with trusting (see the discussion of tend and befriend in Chapter 1) but is still very much part of stress physiology.

1. _____

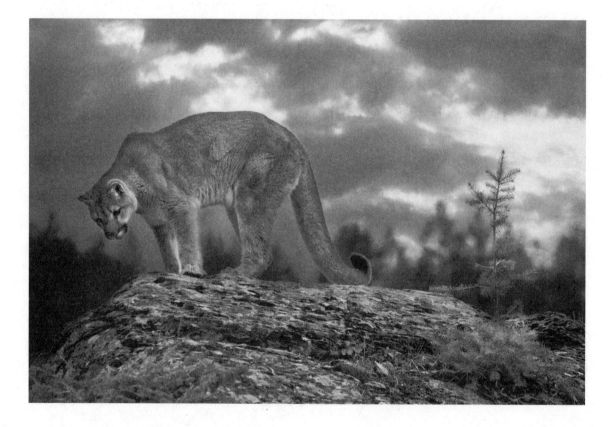

EXERCISE **3.2**

Immediate, Intermediate, and Prolonged Stress Effects

As noted in Chapter 3, the stress response has immediate (seconds), intermediate (minutes to hours), and prolonged (days) effects through which the symptoms of physical stress can manifest. To reinforce your understanding of each phase of this physiological process, please take a moment to reflect on how your body reacts to stress through these three processes.

1. What do you feel when immediately threatened?
   a. Tingling sensations   Yes   No
   b. Sweating   Yes   No
   c. Muscle tension (e.g., jaw muscles)   Yes   No
   d. Rapid heart rate   Yes   No
   e. Rapid breathing (or holding your breath)   Yes   No
   f. Rush of blood to your face and neck (blushing) Yes   No

   g. Other _____

2. How would you best classify your body's intermediate (within hours) response to stress?
   a. Tension headache   Yes   No
   b. Migraine headache   Yes   No
   c. Sore neck and shoulders   Yes   No
   d. Sore throat   Yes   No
   e. Allergies   Yes   No
   f. Stomachache   Yes   No
   g. GI tract problems   Yes   No

   h. Other _____

   i. Other _____

   j. Other _____

   k. Other _____

3. What do you notice as long-term effects of prolonged stress (five to ten days)?

   a. Cold or flu   Yes   No

   b. Acne (broken-out face blemishes)   Yes   No

   c. Herpes flare-up (around lips)   Yes   No

   d. Menstrual period irregularities   Yes   No

   e. Other _____

   f. Other _____

   g. Other _____

   h. Other _____

Stress and Disease

EXERCISE **4.1**

Physical Symptoms Questionnaire

Please look over this list of stress-related symptoms and circle how often they have occurred in the past week, how severe they seemed to you, and how long they lasted. Then reflect on the past week's workload and see whether you notice any connection between your stress levels and possible stress-related symptoms.

		How Often? (Number of days in the past week)	How Severe? (1 = mild; 5 = severe)	How Long? (1 = 1 hour; 5 = all day)
1.	Tension headache	0 1 2 3 4 5 6 7	1 2 3 4 5	1 2 3 4 5
2.	Migraine headache	0 1 2 3 4 5 6 7	1 2 3 4 5	1 2 3 4 5
3.	Muscle tension (neck and/or shoulders)	0 1 2 3 4 5 6 7	1 2 3 4 5	1 2 3 4 5
4.	Muscle tension (lower back)	0 1 2 3 4 5 6 7	1 2 3 4 5	1 2 3 4 5
5.	Joint pain	0 1 2 3 4 5 6 7	1 2 3 4 5	1 2 3 4 5
6.	Cold	0 1 2 3 4 5 6 7	1 2 3 4 5	1 2 3 4 5
7.	Flu	0 1 2 3 4 5 6 7	1 2 3 4 5	1 2 3 4 5
8.	Stomachache	0 1 2 3 4 5 6 7	1 2 3 4 5	1 2 3 4 5
9.	Stomach/abdominal bloating/distention/gas	0 1 2 3 4 5 6 7	1 2 3 4 5	1 2 3 4 5
10.	Diarrhea	0 1 2 3 4 5 6 7	1 2 3 4 5	1 2 3 4 5
11.	Constipation	0 1 2 3 4 5 6 7	1 2 3 4 5	1 2 3 4 5
12.	Ulcer flare-up	0 1 2 3 4 5 6 7	1 2 3 4 5	1 2 3 4 5
13.	Asthma attack	0 1 2 3 4 5 6 7	1 2 3 4 5	1 2 3 4 5
14.	Allergies	0 1 2 3 4 5 6 7	1 2 3 4 5	1 2 3 4 5
15.	Canker/cold sores	0 1 2 3 4 5 6 7	1 2 3 4 5	1 2 3 4 5
16.	Dizzy spells	0 1 2 3 4 5 6 7	1 2 3 4 5	1 2 3 4 5
17.	Heart palpitations (racing heart)	0 1 2 3 4 5 6 7	1 2 3 4 5	1 2 3 4 5
18.	Temporomandibular joint dysfunction (TMJD)	0 1 2 3 4 5 6 7	1 2 3 4 5	1 2 3 4 5

	How Often? (Number of days in the past week)	How Severe? (1 = mild; 5 = severe)	How Long? (1 = 1 hour; 5 = all day)
19. Insomnia	0 1 2 3 4 5 6 7	1 2 3 4 5	1 2 3 4 5
20. Nightmares	0 1 2 3 4 5 6 7	1 2 3 4 5	1 2 3 4 5
21. Fatigue	0 1 2 3 4 5 6 7	1 2 3 4 5	1 2 3 4 5
22. Hemorrhoids	0 1 2 3 4 5 6 7	1 2 3 4 5	1 2 3 4 5
23. Pimples/acne	0 1 2 3 4 5 6 7	1 2 3 4 5	1 2 3 4 5
24. Cramps	0 1 2 3 4 5 6 7	1 2 3 4 5	1 2 3 4 5
25. Frequent accidents	0 1 2 3 4 5 6 7	1 2 3 4 5	1 2 3 4 5
26. Other	0 1 2 3 4 5 6 7	1 2 3 4 5	1 2 3 4 5

(Please specify: _____)

Score: Look over this entire list. Do you observe any patterns or relationships between your stress levels and your physical health? A value over 30 points most likely indicates a stress-related health problem. If it seems to you that these symptoms are related to undue stress, they probably are. Although medical treatment is advocated when necessary, the regular use of relaxation techniques may lessen the intensity, frequency, and duration of these episodes.

Comments:

_____

_____

_____

_____

_____

_____

_____

_____

_____

_____

_____

EXERCISE **4.2**

Your Picture of Health

We all have an idea of what ideal health is. Many of us take our health for granted until something goes wrong. Then we are reminded that our picture of health is compromised and less than ideal. Although health may seem to be objective, it will certainly vary from person to person. It will also vary within each individual over the entire aging process. The following statements are based on characteristics associated with longevity and a healthy quality of life (none of which considers any genetic factors). Rather than answering the questions to see how long you may might live, please complete this inventory to determine your current picture of health.

| 3 = Often | 2 = Sometimes | 1 = Rarely | 0 = Never |

1. With rare exception, I sleep an average of seven to eight hours each night.	3	2	1	0
2. I tend to eat my meals at the same time each day.	3	2	1	0
3. I keep my bedtime consistent every night.	3	2	1	0
4. I do cardiovascular exercise at least three times per week.	3	2	1	0
5. My weight is considered ideal for my height.	3	2	1	0
6. Without exception, my alcohol consumption is moderate.	3	2	1	0
7. I consider my nutritional habits to be exceptional.	3	2	1	0
8. My health status is considered excellent, with no pre-existing conditions.	3	2	1	0
9. I neither smoke nor participate in the use of recreational drugs.	3	2	1	0
10. I have a solid group of friends with whom I socialize regularly.	3	2	1	0

Total score _____

Scoring Key

26–30 points = Excellent health habits
20–25 points = Moderate health habits
14–19 points = Questionable health habits
0–13 points = Poor health habits

EXERCISE **4.3**

My Health Profile

Health is so much more than the optimal functioning of our physical bodies. By and large, however, the physical body is what people focus on when they talk about health (weight, skin, hair, sight, hearing, etc.). To fully understand the mind-body-spirit connection, you must realize that the body is actually the endpoint where unresolved issues of mind and spirit collect, not the beginning. But *if* we were to start with the body and examine, from head to toe, our physical makeup, perhaps we could use this as a stepping stone toward understanding this unique relationship.

Several aspects of our physical makeup, when looked at as a composite, tend to give us a sound understanding of our physical health status. This journal theme invites you to take some time to explore your overall physical health. Once you have compiled all your personal health data, compare your values with the norms discussed in class, or in the book *Managing Stress*. If you have any questions regarding your profile, bring these to the attention of your physician.

My Health Profile

Name _____

Height _____

Weight _____

Age _____

Resting heart rate _____

Target heart rate _____

Maximal heart rate _____

Resting systolic blood pressure _____

Resting diastolic blood pressure _____

Total cholesterol _____

HDL level _____

LDL level _____

Vision status _____

Dental status _____

Hearing status _____

Skin condition _____

Gastrointestinal (GI) tract _____

Tense areas, muscular _____

Reproductive system _____

Skin _____

Sinuses _____

Other _____

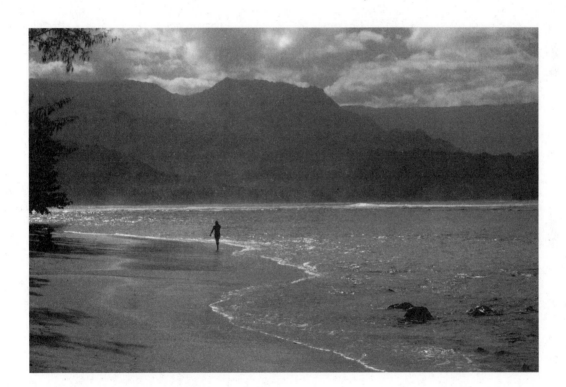

EXERCISE **4.4**

Subtle Anatomy Energy Map

The accompanying figure is an outline of the human body with the seven primary chakras highlighted. The first chakra is called the base chakra and the seventh chakra is called the crown chakra (also known as the halo). Note the body region associated with each chakra, as well as the aspects with which each chakra is associated, and then take a moment to identify any health issues or concerns associated with this specific region of your body. Once you have done this, ask yourself honestly whether you recognize any connection between the important aspects of the chakra(s) associated with the region(s) that you have indicated and a specific health concern.

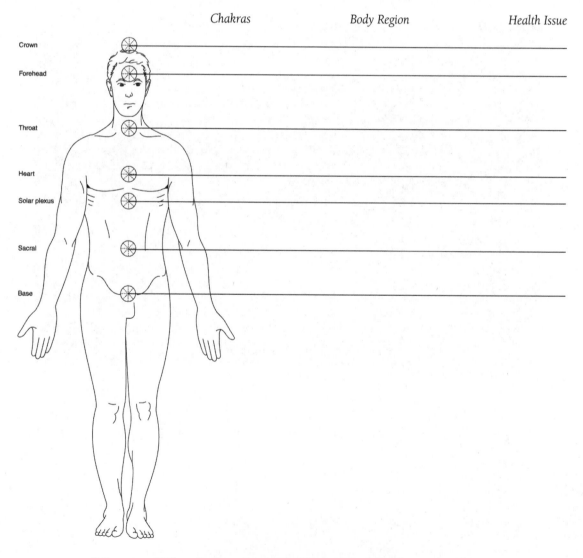

EXERCISE **4.5**

When Your Biography Becomes Your Biology

The cause of illness is ultimately connected to the inner stresses present in a person's life.
Caroline Myss

In the early 1980s, Robert Ader coined the term *psychoneuroimmunology* to distinguish a new field of study, the field of mind-body medicine. What he and now countless others have discovered is that there is an amazing and profound connection between the mind, body, and spirit. Contrary to French philosopher Renée Descartes' reductionistic theory, the mind and body are not separate entities. This means that our minds and the emotional thoughts we produce have an incredible impact on our physiology, for better or worse.

One person who has emerged in the forefront of mind-body medicine is Caroline Myss, PhD. A woman with an incredible ability to see what most others cannot, Myss can view a person's energy field and assist physicians in determining the onset and location of disease as well as the cause of a disease. Myss has a remarkable rate of accuracy, especially considering that she can do this from hundreds of miles away (known as non-local viewing or medical intuition). First intrigued by the concepts of the human energy field and the chakras (spinning wheels of energy positioned over several major body organs from head to spine), Myss has focused her own energy into teaching people awareness of mind-body-spirit harmony.

In one of her first books, *The Creation of Health*, Myss discusses the idea that a life history, in terms of experiences, becomes intertwined with the cells of our physical bodies (Shealy and Myss, 1988). From hundreds of documented case studies, she has come to the understanding that symptoms of disease and illness don't start in the body; they end there. Can cervical cancer be rooted in sexual molestation? Can lower back pain be rooted in financial insecurities? Can bone spurs on the heel of the foot be a result of feeling "defeated"? Myss thinks so. Judging by her track record (95 percent accuracy of diagnosing diseases), she stands on pretty solid ground.

According to Caroline Myss, getting your life story out and examined is one of the first steps toward optimal health. By coming to terms with your biography, you can release the negative energies that distort the integrity of each and every cell in your body. So what is your biography? What are some of the most significant (perhaps emotionally painful) events that you now carry in the memory of each cell? Take some time to explore these and perhaps other lifelong memories that may now be a part of your biology.

_____

_____

_____

_____

35

EXERCISE **4.6**

Energy Ball Exercise

This relaxation technique was taught to me by the renowned bio-energy healers Mietek and Margaret Wirkus. I have adapted and taught this technique many times in classes and workshops throughout the country, with great success. Although it was introduced to me as the first of many healing techniques in bio-energy healing, first and foremost it is a relaxation exercise. This technique is done through the following steps.

1. Begin by sitting comfortably with your legs crossed and your back straight. You may wish to sit up against a wall. In this exercise, it really helps to keep your back straight. Close your eyes and focus your attention on your breathing. Take a moment to clear your mind of distracting thoughts and feelings. Place your attention on your breathing. If it helps to have some soft instrumental music in the background, then try this as well. Sometimes, to set the tone, it helps to think of a happy moment in your life, when you were filled with utter joy. Allow this feeling to resonate within every cell in your body. Then take a couple of comfortably slow, deep breaths to let the feeling be absorbed.

2. Unlike the belly breathing technique that is typically taught in relaxation workshops, this particular exercise requires that you focus your attention on the upper lobes of your lungs. Take a moment to place your hands on your upper chest to become fully conscious of your upper lungs. Then take five breaths, breathing comfortably slow and deep into your upper lungs.

3. Once you have completed this, place your hands on your knees and repeat this breathing style by taking five slow, deep breaths. As you exhale, repeat this phrase to yourself: "My body is calm and relaxed." As you say this, feel a deep sense of relaxation throughout your body with each exhalation.

4. Next, being fully conscious of your hands resting on your knees or thighs, take five more deep breaths, but this time as you exhale, repeat this phrase to yourself: "I am my hands." With each breath, place all of your concentration, all of your attention, on your hands. Sense what your hands feel like. Are they warm? If so, where? On the palms, fingertips, the backs of your hands? Again, remind yourself of the phrase, "I am my hands."

5. Using your imagination, picture a small window in the center of each palm, about the size of a dime. Imagine now that as you breathe, air not only comes into your nose or mouth, but into your hands as well. If you prefer, you may use the image of light coming into your palms. Imagine that as you inhale, air or light enters your palms and moves up your arms, to the center (heart space) of your upper chest. As you exhale, feel the energy return from where it entered through your hands. Try repeating this several times, again taking several slow, deep breaths and repeating to yourself, "I am my hands."

6. Next, slowly lift your hands off your knees or thighs so that they rest comfortably in the air, suspended in front of your chest, with the palms facing up, toward the ceiling.

7. Next, fully conscious of your hands, take five more deep breaths. As you exhale each breath, repeat the phrase, "I am my hands." With each breath, place all of your concentration, all of your attention, on your hands. Again sense what your hands feel like. Are they warm? If so, where? On the palms, the fingertips, the backs of your hands? Do your hands feel heavy? If so, how heavy? What other sensations do you feel? Again remind yourself as you exhale, "I am my hands." As you do this, notice whether you see any colors.

8. Now, keeping your hands about ten to twelve inches apart, allow the palms of your hands to face each other. Again using your imagination, picture or sense that between your hands is a large sponge ball. As you hold this ball, slowly press in and then release. What do you feel as you do this? Again, bring your hands closer together without touching, then begin to move them farther apart. Ask yourself what you feel. At what distance is the sensation the strongest?

9. Now, placing the palms of your hands about six to twelve inches apart, imagine that there is a beam of light from palm to palm, window to window. Take a slow, deep breath and as you exhale, slowly compress the beam by bringing your palms together without touching. Then, during the next inhalation, allow your hands to separate again slowly. What do you feel as you do this? Is the sensation between your hands stronger when you inhale or exhale?

10. Again, return to the sensation between your hands. Between your hands is a ball of energy, the healing energy ball. Take this ball of energy and place it in a region of your body that feels stressed or desires healing. If you are completely relaxed, try placing this energy in your heart. Take five slow, deep breaths and repeat the phrase, "My body is calm and relaxed." Feel a sense of relaxation throughout your entire body. Take one final slow, deep breath and enjoy this sensation again.

11. When you are done, slowly place your hands back on your knees or thighs. Recognize that although you feel relaxed, you also feel energized. When you are ready, open your eyes to a soft gaze in front of you. Then make yourself aware of your surroundings so that you may continue on with your daily activities.

Your Experience

Please take a few minutes to describe your experience here:

_____

_____

_____

_____

_____

_____

EXERCISE **4.7**

Subtle Energy System "Vitamins"

Donna Eden is a renowned energy healer with a gift not only for observing subtle energies, but also for teaching others how to regulate their subtle energy for enhanced health and well-being. Integrating the flow of energy through the human aura, chakras, and meridians, Donna combines a variety of self-help techniques so that, in her words, "You keep your energies humming and vibrant." The following are energy exercises that Donna teaches in her energy medicine workshops, exercises that she calls "energy system vitamins." She recommends that you do this short routine daily to keep your immune system at an optimal level.

1. **Three body taps.** There are various acupuncture/acupressure points that, when stimulated, will help direct the flow of energy, and thus increase your vitality and help boost your immune system.

   - *Chestbone tap:* This point is known to acupuncturists as K27 (from points on the kidney meridian). Gently tap on the top of your chest bone just below where the two clavicles meet for about fifteen to twenty seconds, using the fingertips of both hands.

   - *Thymus gland tap:* Your thymus gland (an important gland of the immune system) resides between your throat and your heart, but the point to tap is in the center of your chest, about two inches below K27. Once you have found this point, tap on it with your fingertips for about fifteen to twenty seconds.

   - *Spleen points tap:* The spleen is also an essential organ of your immune system. The spleen points are located on the rib cage, directly below your nipples. Once you have found these two points, tap vigorously with your fingers for about fifteen to twenty seconds.

2. **Cross crawl movements.** To do the cross crawl, first you must understand that the left side of the brain controls the right side of the body, and vice versa. Many people's energies are not vibrant or harmonized because of stagnation; that is, the lack of neural energy moving from the right to left or left to right sides of the brain. Poor energy movement is referred to as a homo-lateral pattern; this will affect thought processes, coordination, and vitality. Sitting or standing, raise your right knee and your left arm (you can touch knee to elbow if you'd like). Follow this by raising your left knee and your right arm. Twist your torso so that your arms cross the mid-point of your body. Try this movement pattern for about thirty to sixty seconds.

3. **The crown pull.** Placing your hand on top of your forehead and crown of the head, imagine that your fingers are pulling from the center down to your ears, in a motion starting from the front of your head and working to the back of your skull. The purpose of this exercise is to move stagnant energy from the top of your head and help to open the crown chakra. This exercise can be helpful in relieving headaches, too.

4. **Zip up.** The central meridian (in the front of your body) can easily become congested, open, or exposed to others' energy. This technique invites you to close your auric field as a means of health and protection. Start by tapping the K27 point again and then reach down to the top of your thighs with your right (or left) hand, take a deep breath, and pull up as if you were pulling up a zipper, clear up to your chin. Repeat this three times. By pulling up, you trace the directional flow of the central meridian and strengthen the flow of energy. This technique is recommended before making speeches or dealing with someone who is very angry.

After having practiced these energy vitamins for several days, what is your experience with health status? Have you noticed a difference in your levels of personal energy? How is your energy status vital?

_____

_____

_____

_____

_____

_____

_____

_____

_____

_____

_____

_____

_____

_____

_____

_____

_____

The Mind and the Soul

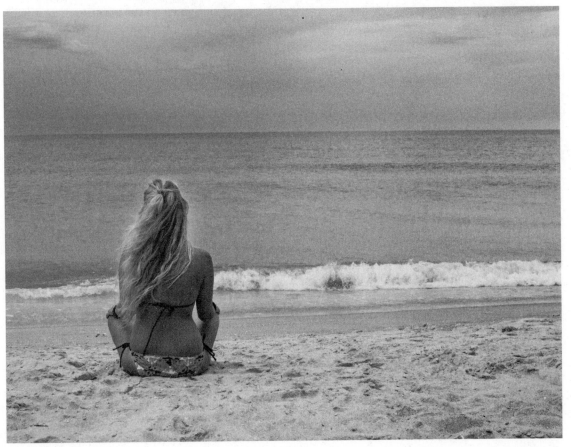

Toward a Psychology of Stress

EXERCISE **5.1**

The Psychology of Your Stress

The following questions are based on several theories from Chapter 5 to help you become more aware of your perceptions, attitudes, and behaviors during episodes of stress:

1. In hindsight (because Freud said people are not aware at the time that they are doing it), do you find that you use one or more defense mechanisms to protect your ego? Reflecting on your behavior, which of the following do you see as common behaviors in your psychology of stress profile?

   a. Defensiveness (I didn't do it)   Yes   (No)

   b. Projection (She did it)   (Yes)   No

   c. Repression (I don't remember doing it)   (Yes)   No

   d. Displacement (He made me do it)   Yes   (No)

   e. Rationalization (Everyone does it)   Yes   (No)

   f. Humor (I can laugh about this now)   (Yes)   No

   g. Other _____

2. Carl Jung was adamant that we need to listen to the wisdom of our dreams. Please answer the following questions based on Jung's theories related to stress.

   a. Do you often remember your dreams?   Yes   (No)

   b. Do you make it a habit to try to understand your dreams
      and dream symbols?   Yes   (No)

   c. Do you have any recurring dreams?   Yes   (No)

   d. Have you ever had a dream of an event that later came
      to pass?   (Yes)   No

3. Kübler-Ross's stages of grieving are not just for cancer patients. These same stages occur for the death of every unmet expectation. What recent expectation was unmet that brought you to the door of the grieving process? What stage of Kübler-Ross's progression have you currently reached with this stressor?

Leaving my IP job → feeling I could no longer be effective

ANGER, still

4. Refer to Exercise 1.5 ("Personal Stress Inventory: Top Ten Stressors"). If it has been a while since you have looked at this list, please consider updating it. After having done this, please list your stressors as predominantly anger-based or fear-based stressors.

Anger-Based Stressors

a. *finances - debt*

b. *job change*

c. _____

Fear-Based Stressors

a. *my uncle's stroke*

b. *aunt's cancer*

c. _____

EXERCISE **5.2**

Domestication of the Ego

Where there is stress, there's ego.
Deepak Chopra

Renowned psychologist Carl Jung once said, "The conscious mind rejects that which it does not understand." What he meant by that statement is that the ego acts as a powerful censor to the wealth of information residing just below the surface of conscious thought. Not only does the ego *not* make an attempt to understand the unconscious mind, it reacts to all unfamiliar ideas as enemies at the gate, ready to be shot down on a mere whim. Like an oversensitive security system that activates at the hint of a threat, the ego defends us not only against real danger but also against illusionary dangers that it creates itself. The net result is that we lose out on a lot in life by having an overprotective ego, one always trying to maintain control rather than empowering us to new heights.

In Eastern culture, there is an expression that reminds us to beware of an overprotective ego. It is said that we need to learn to "domesticate our ego" or else run the risk of having "poop" all over the place. What can one do to start this domestication process? First, you have to admit that, indeed, your ego can be the source of problems; if nothing else, it holds you back and limits your human potential. To do this, you have to observe your thought processes on a regular basis, repeatedly catch yourself in the act, and stop this limiting ego process in midstream enough times so that this new behavior takes root, becomes second nature, and replaces the old and useless thought processes of an overreactive and self-defeating ego.

Carl Jung often used the phrase "embracing the shadow," an expression he is credited with coining to represent the dark side of the ego. But before you embrace (versus exploit) your dark side, you must first tame it by being conscious of thoughts that are fear based.

Domesticating the ego requires more than easing up on the suppressing role of the censor. It also means not viewing people, things, and opportunities as threats to one's existence. Furthermore, it means engaging in acts of forgiveness, tolerance, patience, and compassion.

The following are some questions to ponder about things that might push your buttons but, with a little bit of thought, might also allow you to housetrain your ego.

1. What types of people do you feel a sense of prejudice toward or against? List them here, and next to each answer write a short explanation of why you harbor these feelings.

   a. _____

   b. _____

   c. _____

2. What stereotypes do you find yourself labeling people with? What is the basis for these thoughts?

   a. _____

   b. _____

   c. _____

3. Name three people you find yourself trying to control or manipulate:

   a. _____

   b. _____

   c. _____

4. If you had to list three insecurities you have, what would you identify?

   a. _____

   b. _____

   c. _____

5. Describe in a few words your most common recurring dream:

   _____

   _____

   _____

6. List three of the deepest fears that you can identify (please be specific).

   a. _____

   b. _____

   c. _____

7. What three people are you holding grudges against? Next to each name, write how long you have been nurturing this sense of resentment and why the grudge still exists.

   a. _____

   b. _____

   c. _____

8. Additional thoughts: _____

   _____

   _____

EXERCISE **5.3**

Fifteen Minutes of Fame

Almost everybody wants to be famous. Why? We all like recognition, and we crave acceptance. Even people who consider themselves introverts like to be considered worthy by their family, friends, and peers. In this age of high technology, the chance of becoming famous is increasing dramatically; it seems as if everybody has his or her own television show and Web site or YouTube video these days. But fame never lasts long. With rare exceptions, fame evaporates more quickly than a cup of water in the desert sun. When one face disappears, a new one comes along immediately. Fame is nothing more than the ego revealed.

Renowned artist Andy Warhol once said that everybody wants his or her 15 minutes of fame. What he meant was that everyone craves acceptance, and many people desire notoriety. Nowhere is this more evident than reality TV shows and YouTube videos where people are clamoring to get noticed. Perhaps it's because American culture projects a sense of high esteem for those people who have "made it." When you consider what movie actors and professional athletes get paid compared with what schoolteachers earn, it becomes clear that fame and fortune *are* American values. Perhaps the real questions are, What is success? And why do we seek pleasure through media venues?

The concept of 15 minutes of fame speaks to more than just the concept of being famous. It really speaks to the concept of ego. Freud is given credit for coining the term *ego*, but in fact the concept of being self-centered is as old as humanity itself. Freud said that the purpose of ego is to provide pleasure and minimize pain. As bad or big as some egos appear, the truth is, we all need an ego. Our egos serve as our bodyguards. The trouble is that with a great many people, the bodyguard wants a promotion and a new job title (e.g., *the* boss).

This journal theme is about ego. Here are some questions to ponder:

1. On a scale of 1 to 10 (with 1 being low), how would you rate the strength of your ego?

2. Do you think egotistical behavior is genetic or a learned behavior? Why?

3. In your opinion, how does ego relate to self-esteem?

4. Do you ever crave acceptance, notoriety, or fame? Why do you suppose this is so? How much of this is influenced by television, magazines, and so on?

5. There is an expression used in Eastern culture: "Domesticate the ego, or you'll have poop all over the place." What are some ways in which you can domesticate your ego and still maintain your self-esteem?

6. Any other comments you wish to share here before you step into the limelight?

_____

_____

_____

EXERCISE **5.4**

Dreams: The Language of Symbols

Dreams are a powerful language. They offer insight into the shadows and depths of our unconscious mind. Carl Jung, world-renowned psychologist and a pioneer in dream analysis, stated that dreams offer a basis of psychic balance—if only we would take the time to become more aware of them and reflect on their meaning. Although often expressed in a language of symbols, dreams may offer insight into ways to resolve our current problems. This insight begins with an awareness of dream fragments, followed by an interpretation process. As Jung suggested, the dream cannot be separated from the dreamer, and indeed, each of us is best suited to interpret our own dreams. A full interpretation, however, comes from looking at the dream image from every perspective to try to understand its meaning.

To enhance this awareness of dreams, try leaving your journal by your nightstand and remind yourself before you fall asleep that you want to remember your dreams. Upon first waking, record whatever dream images or fragments you can recall. Then mull over these images and listen to the thoughts they suggest. You may wish to revisit these dream images because their meaning is not always obvious. Experts agree that not all dreams are significant, but the act of recording your images from the dream state may help you to deal more effectively with concerns and issues that you confront in your waking hours.

What recent dream do you recall that seemed significant? Do any objects that you recall seem to offer personal symbolism? After thinking about the fragments or sequences, do they begin to make any sense to you? Please write your thoughts down here.

_____

_____

_____

_____

_____

_____

_____

_____

_____

EXERCISE **5.5**

Dreams Revisited

Although we all have dreams, remembering them is not always easy. But there are occasions when a certain dream is replayed in our mind over the course of months, perhaps even years. These recurring dreams may only have a short run on the mind's silver screen (e.g., seconds), or they may last throughout our lifetime. These dreams, perhaps foggy in detail, surface occasionally in the conscious state, and the story they tell is all too familiar: Some issue is begging for resolution.

It is commonly believed that recurring dreams symbolize a hidden insecurity or a stressful event that has yet to be resolved. Simply stated, they don't have resolved endings (e.g., you wake up, sometimes out of sheer panic, before the story in the dream ends). While there is much to the dream state that is still unknown, it is believed that dreams are images that the unconscious mind creates to communicate to the conscious mind in a language all its own. This form of communication is not a one-way street. Messages can be sent to the unconscious mind in a normal waking state as well.

Through the use of mental imagery, you can script the final scenes of a recurring dream with a happy ending. What seems to be the final scene of a dream is actually the beginning of the resolution process. The following is a true story: Once there was a young boy who had an afternoon paper route. One day while the boy was delivering papers, a large black German shepherd jumped out of the bushes and attacked him. The owner called the dog back, but not before the dog drew blood. As the boy grew into adulthood, his love for dogs never diminished, but several times a year he awoke in a sweat from a recurring dream he had had once too often. *The dream:* "It is dark and I am walking through the woods at night. Out from behind one of the trees comes this huge black dog. All I can see are his teeth, and all I can hear is his bark. I try to yell for help, but nothing comes out of my throat. Just as he lunges for me, I awake in a panic."

With a little thought and imagination, a final scene was drafted to bring closure to this dream story. *Final scene:* "I am walking through the woods at night with a flashlight, a bone, and a can of mace. This time when the dog lunges at me, I shine the light in his eyes and spray mace in his face. He whines and whines, and then I tell him to sit. He obeys. I put the bone by his nose and he looks at me inquisitively. Then he licks the bone and starts to bite into it. I begin to walk away and the dog gets up to follow, bone in mouth. I stop and look back and he stops. He wags his tail. The sky grows light as the sun begins to rise, and the black night fades into pink and orange clouds. As I walk back to my house, I see the dog take his new find down the street. I open the door and walk upstairs and crawl back into bed." It has been five years, and this man has never had this dream again.

Ultimately we are the creators of our dreams. We are the writers, directors, producers, and actors of our dreams. Although drafting a final scene is no guarantee that the issues that produce recurring dreams will be resolved, it is a great starting point in the resolution process, a time for reflection that may open up the channels of communication between the conscious and unconscious minds. In fact, in most cases, the active imaginative process of completing recurring dreams sets things in motion for resolution. Do you have a recurring dream that needs a final scene to be complete? Write out your recurring dream and give it a final scene.

EXERCISE **5.6**

Guilt and Worry

The difference between a state of stress and a state of relaxation is simple. In a stressful frame of mind, we are preoccupied with events or issues from the past or the future, or both. In a state of relaxation, we can enjoy the present moment; we can absorb and appreciate life's simple pleasures. Stress robs us of the present moment.

As psychologist Wayne Dyer suggests in his best-selling book *Your Erroneous Zones*, two human emotions are employed exclusively in the stressful state of mind: guilt and worry. *Guilt* preoccupies the mind with events and feelings from the past, whereas *worry* focuses our attention on anticipated events. What both of these emotional states, or zones, have in common is that they immobilize our thought processes and leave us unable to function at our best. These emotions cloud the mind and freeze rational thought processes that are truly needed to deal with our stressors.

Although events from our past may serve as excellent learning experiences, all the guilt in the world will not change what has already occurred. Likewise, worrying is unproductive thinking. Too much of it can wreak havoc with the body's internal organs. Worrying about the future (not to be confused with planning for the future) is an unproductive emotion. Worrying is an immobilizing emotion. It wastes a lot of time, and time is too valuable a resource to waste. Most, if not all, of our stressors produce an excess of either one or both of these emotions. Not only do they rob us of the ability to enjoy the present moment, but they also inhibit us from acting in a way to resolve the issue that created these emotional responses.

Are you a chronic worrier? Are there specific times that you fret about, or do general concerns trigger your worries? Make a list of your top ten stressors again. Take a good look at them. Do they promote guilt or worry? Many people feel uncomfortable in the present moment. They would rather focus their attention on past or future events to avoid the present moment. Are you one of these people? Self-imposed guilt trips are very stressful. Is this an occasional characteristic of yours? Do you lay an occasional guilt trip on others to manipulate their emotions and behavior? If so, why? What are some ways to cut down the use of these two emotions in your strategy to deal effectively with stress?

EXERCISE **5.7**

All You Need Is Love

Love means letting go of fear.
Gerald Jampolski

Love. It seems that no other concept has puzzled humankind so much as this. It is love that gives life, and paradoxically, people lose their lives in the name of love. As a professor who studied, taught, and has written several books on the subject, Dr. Leo Buscaglia admits that to define love is virtually impossible. Impossible it may be, but like pursuing the elusive Holy Grail, people continue to try. Among authors, poets, songwriters, and actors, the vehicles of love's message are endless.

After years of research and personal insight, Buscaglia offered his own incomplete definition, suggesting that love is that which brings you back to your real self. In Buscaglia's book entitled *Love*, he writes, "For love and the self are one and the discovery of either is the realization of both." Just as charity is said to begin at home, so too must love reside within the individual before it can be shared. Buscaglia notes that the ability to feel and express love of the self is literally frowned upon as being selfish. In reality, he suggests that to share love you must first give yourself permission to possess and nurture this quality within yourself. Furthermore, self-love begins with self-acceptance, unconditional self-acceptance.

It is interesting to note that the field of psychology has pretty much ignored this emotion during the twentieth century, instead giving the limelight to anxiety and fear. Because of sexual connotations, love as an inner resource has been virtually disregarded, much to the detriment of all human society. More recently, this aspect of the human condition has been given more serious attention. In the much-acclaimed book *The Road Less Traveled*, psychiatrist M. Scott Peck offers his insights about love. From empirical observations, Peck perceived that there are many echelons of love: sharing, caring, trust, passion, and compassion, with the highest level of love being a divine essence he calls *grace*.

Let there be no doubt, love is a profound concept. It is a value, an emotion, a virtue, a spiritual essence, an energy, and, to many people, an enigma. Love can inflict emotional pain, just as it can heal the scars and bruises of the soul. It can make a fool out of the bravest man and a hero out of an underdog. The expression of love can be quite intimidating as well, and in American society, love is often extended with conditions. Ultimately, such strings taint our perception of love, whereas unconditional love may be the ultimate expression of grace. When people hear the word *love*, visions of Hollywood silver-screen passion come to mind. We have been socialized to think that love has to be as dynamic as Superman, yet the power of love can be as subtle as a smile or a happy thought. There are many colors in love's rainbow.

If you were to make an attempt to define love, how would you begin to describe your interpretation of this concept? Is your expression of love limited by your level of self-acceptance? In your expression of love to others, do you find that you attach conditions? In your opinion, how does falling in love differ from unconditional love? Add any thoughts to your definition of love here.

EXERCISE **5.8**

Creative Altruism: The Power of Unconditional Love

Love, it is said, is the glue that holds the universe together. The expression of love can be made manifest in a great many ways. The following questions encourage you to explore the concept of unconditional love as an alternative to the motivation of fear.

1. Write your best definition of love:

   _____

   _____

2. If love is the energy that moves the human spirit, then fear is the metaphorical brake that stops love in its tracks. How does fear impede your ability to express love?

   _____

   _____

3. The slogan "Perform random acts of kindness" was coined by a woman who was searching for a way to make the world a better place in which to live. She created this catch phrase as a means to express heartfelt altruism. Performing a random act of kindness means giving anonymously without the expectation of receiving anything in return. Compose a list of five ways to "give" altruistically and identify at least three ways that don't involve money.

   a. _____

   b. _____

   c. _____

   d. _____

   e. _____

4. Service! One cannot speak on the topic of altruism without speaking of the concept of service, yet service is an idea that has fallen on deaf ears lately. It's hard to feel sorry for yourself when you are helping others who are less fortunate. Over the past decade, the Institute of Noetic Sciences has given the Creative Altruism Award to those unique individuals who demonstrate the spirit of selfless

service. If you could create an altruistic nonprofit organization to help others, what would you do? Explain it here:

_____

_____

_____

_____

_____

_____

_____

_____

_____

_____

_____

_____

_____

_____

_____

_____

_____

_____

_____

_____

_____

EXERCISE **5.9**

Mind over Matter: Harnessing the Power of Your Mind

Spoon bending may seem to be in a different league than the spontaneous remission of a cancerous tumor, but in reality, the premise of each is the same. Most likely you've heard the expression "mind over matter," yet few people actually put this philosophy into play. Mind over matter simply means using the power of your mind (both conscious and unconscious minds) to accomplish a task. Mind over matter isn't a means of controlling others. Rather, it's a means of becoming empowered instead of giving your power away. Those who teach mind power often use the spoon-bending exercise as the first stepping stone toward the goal of other, seemingly larger but no less challenging goals. Mind over matter isn't magic, an illusion, or a cute parlor trick. It's merely the manifestation of an inherent power that we each hold in the center of our own minds. The process of mind over matter involves the following three distinct steps.

- **Step 1: Focus your mind.** The first step of the process requires your mind to be focused completely and entirely on the task at hand. A wandering mind is analogous to irritating static on your favorite radio station making the transmission inaudible.

- **Step 2: Believe.** Once the mind is clear of distracting thoughts and is completely focused on the task at hand, the heart and mind (conscious and unconscious minds) must be aligned. This means that all doubt must be cast aside, and faith must galvanize you with a sense of absolutely knowing that you will, indeed, accomplish the deed (whatever it happens to be). To reinforce the belief process, use the power of your imagination to picture the event as having already occurred. Feel the exhilaration of completing this task.

- **Step 3: State the command.** State the command to complete the desired action. To bend a spoon, you might simply state, "Bend!" To dissolve a tumor, state the command, "Dissolve away!"

Spoon Bending 101

Locate an old spoon (or fork) from the silverware drawer (one that you don't intend to use again). Hold the base of the utensil in one hand and with a slight effort of the free hand apply a little pressure simply to test the strength of the metal. Follow steps 1 to 3 (above). After stating the command "Bend!" once again hold the top of the utensil and bend it at the neck. If possible, bend the neck of the spoon or fork into a loop. Remember, this is not an exercise of muscular strength in your fingers, but rather of willpower from the depths of your unconscious mind. Sometimes it helps to visualize the neck of the spoon as molten red right before you apply pressure to bend the spoon. Once the utensil is transformed, consider keeping it in a place where you can see it often as a symbol to remind you of the power of your mind.

Spoon bending is really nothing more than a simple metaphor of the power of mind over matter. Once you have mastered this task, consider trying this technique in other areas of your life.

Describe your experience here:

_____

_____

_____

_____

_____

_____

_____

_____

_____

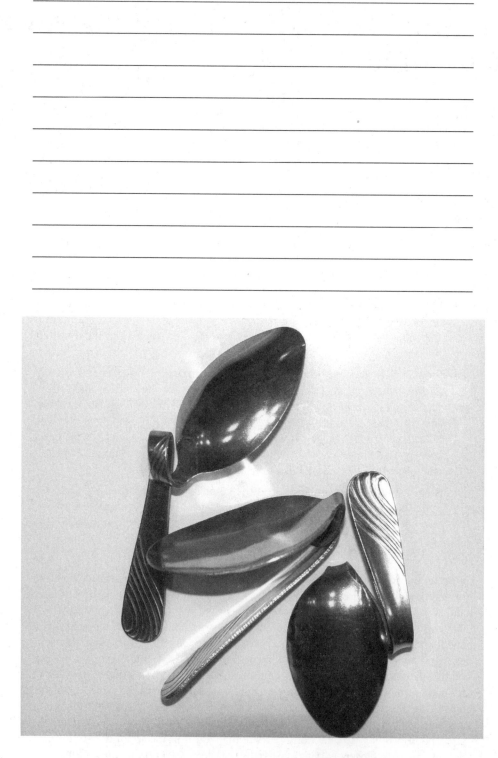

The Stress Emotions: Anger, Fear, and Joy

EXERCISE **6.1**

Anger Recognition Checklist

He who angers you, conquers you.
Elizabeth Kenny

The following is a quick exercise to help you understand how anger can surface in the course of a normal working day and how you *may* mismanage it. Please place a check mark in front of any of the following that apply to you when you get angry or feel frustrated or upset. After completing this section, please refer to the bottom right-hand corner to estimate, on average, the number of episodes of anger you experience per day.

When I feel angry, my anger tends to surface in the following ways:

_____ anxiety	_____ threatening others
_____ depression	_____ buying things
_____ overeating	_____ frequent lateness
_____ starting to diet	_____ I never feel angry
_____ trouble sleeping	_____ clenched jaw muscles, TMJD
_____ excessive sleeping	_____ boredom
_____ careless driving	_____ nausea, vomiting
_____ chronic fatigue	_____ skin problems
_____ abuse of alcohol/drugs	_____ easy irritation
_____ exploding in rage	_____ sexual difficulty
_____ cold withdrawal	_____ sexual apathy
_____ tension headaches	_____ busy work (clean, straighten)
_____ migraine headaches	_____ sulking, whining

_____ use of sarcasm

_____ hostile joking

_____ being accident prone

_____ guilt and self-blame

_____ smoking or drinking

_____ high blood pressure

_____ frequent nightmares

_____ tendency to harp or nag

_____ intellectualization

_____ upset stomach (e.g., gas, cramps, IBS)

_____ muscle tension (neck, lower back)

_____ swearing or name calling

_____ crying

_____ hitting, throwing things

_____ complaining, whining

_____ cutting/mutilating myself

_____ insomnia

_____ promiscuity

_____ helping others

_____ other? _____

_____ other? _____

* My average number of anger episodes per day is _____.

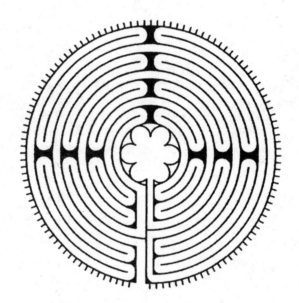

EXERCISE **6.2**

Mismanaged Anger Style Indicator

Part I: Check the statements that are true for you the majority of the time.

_____ 1. Even though I may wish to complain, I usually don't.

_____ 2. When upset, I have a habit of slamming, punching, or breaking things.

_____ 3. When I feel guilty, I have been known to contemplate self-destructive behaviors.

_____ 4. I can be real nice to people, but then backstab them when they're not around.

_____ 5. I have a habit of grinding my teeth at night or tensing my jaw muscles.

_____ 6. When I am really irritated or frustrated by others, I tend to intimidate them.

_____ 7. When I am frustrated, I feel like going shopping and spending money.

_____ 8. I can manipulate people without them even knowing it.

_____ 9. It's fair to say that I rarely, if ever, get angry or mad.

_____ 10. I have been known to talk back to people of authority.

_____ 11. Sleeping in is a good way to forget about my problems and frustrations.

_____ 12. Watching TV or playing video games offers a good escape from my frustrations.

_____ 13. If I complain, I feel people won't like me as much, so I usually don't.

_____ 14. When driving at times, I feel like I want to hit people with my car.

_____ 15. When I get mad or frustrated, I have been known to eat to calm my nerves.

_____ 16. I plan a script or rehearse what I am going to say to win a conflict.

_____ 17. It's hard or uncomfortable for me to say the words "I am angry."

_____ 18. I usually try to get the final say in situations with others.

_____ 19. I have been known to use alcohol and/or drugs to deal with my feelings of anger.

_____ 20. By and large, I tend to agree with the statement "Don't get mad, get even."

_____ 21. I tend to keep my feelings to myself.

_____ 22. When I get angry, I have been known to swear a lot.

_____ 23. I usually feel guilty about feeling angry, frustrated, or annoyed.

_____ 24. It's OK to use sarcasm to make a point.

_____ 25. I am the kind of person who calms the waters when tempers flare at home or work.

_____ 26. It's easy to say the words "I am angry" or "I am pissed" and really mean it.

_____ 27. On more than one occasion, I have imagined taking my own life.

_____ 28. I think of various ways to put people down.

_____ 29. Typically, I place the needs of others before myself.

_____ 30. I suffer from migraine headaches or TMJD or rheumatoid arthritis or lupus.

Once you have completed this survey, please read the score sheet below to best determine which mismanaged anger style is most dominant in your personality. Then please read the detailed descriptions of each style in Exercise 6.3.

Part II: Score Sheet

Write down the numbers of the statements that you checked off in Part I:

_____.

As a rule, we all tend to engage in all of these behaviors at some time; however, some behaviors are very common for us, whereas others are more occasional, suggesting that when certain predominant behaviors are grouped together they will reveal a specific style of mismanaged anger. Mismanaged anger leads to a host of serious problems for both ourselves and others. By learning to recognize series of behaviors that fall into one or perhaps two categories, we can more easily identify this pattern and then make a strategy to change or modify it so that stress is reduced rather than perpetuated. Labels are good for identifying behaviors, but they are not meant to serve as mismanaged scarlet letters.

- If you have four or more answers from choices 1, 5, 9, 13, 17, 21, 25, 29, or 30, your mismanaged anger style strongly suggests you might be a **somatizer (silent but deadly stone)**.

- If you have four or more answers from choices 2, 6, 10, 14, 18, 22, or 26, your mismanaged anger style strongly suggests you might be an **exploder (volcanic stone)**.

- If you have four or more answers from choices 3, 7, 11, 12, 15, 19, 23, or 27, your mismanaged anger style strongly suggests you might be a **self-punisher (razor stone)**.

- If you have four or more answers from choices 4, 8, 16, 20, 24, or 28, your mismanaged anger style strongly suggests you might be an **underhander (revenge stone)**.

EXERCISE **6.3**

The Mismanaged Hot Stones

Anger is like a hot stone. If you pick it up to throw at someone, you will get burned.
Ancient proverb

- **The silent but deadly stone (somatizer).** Some people never seem to get angry. Perhaps, as kids, their parents told them repeatedly, "Don't get mad" or "Don't you ever talk back to me" or "Don't give someone the satisfaction of knowing they hurt you," and so they never do. It's as if they actually swallow these hot stones just to get rid of any trace of anger. It may look as if these people never show feelings of frustration (just a happy face), but what is silence on the surface soon becomes a health problem. In essence, the body becomes the battlefield for the war games of the mind. Examples of health problems associated with this style of unresolved anger are migraine headaches; tension headaches; temporomandibular joint dysfunction, or TMJD (grinding your teeth at night); and digestive problems.

- **The volcanic hot stone (exploder).** When some people get mad, they are like a volcano ready to erupt. Like a volcano, these people seem to have steam coming out of their ears and nostrils. They often use swear words, they may hit something or someone, or they might "flip the bird" at the slightest hint of insult. Some examples of explosive behavior are cursing, verbal intimidation, slamming doors, throwing things, kicking things or people, road rage, sports rage, and physical abuse.

- **The razor stone (self-punisher).** The razor stone is not only hot, but also sharp. First it burns; then it cuts deep. Not only is there frustration associated with this stone, but there is guilt as well—guilt from feeling angry. The kinds of people who hold this hot stone feel so bad about feeling guilty that they engage in some excessive behavior to make themselves feel better. Many eating disorders, such as anorexia and bulimia, fall into this category. Self-mutilation (i.e., cutting) and depression (depression is anger turned inward) are often linked to holding the razor stone. Some other examples of this mismanaged anger are excessive smoking, sleeping, exercise, drinking, drug use, shopping, and playing video games.

- **The revenge hot stone (underhander).** The motto of the person who holds the revenge stone is "Don't get mad; get even." Some people try to get more than even; they get one up. This kind of person seeks revenge by getting even in a passive-aggressive way. In other words, these people are nice to you, but the minute you turn your back, they start hurling the revenge stone. For others, the revenge stone is the "grudge stone." Once again, the holders of this stone may hit their target, but get burned badly in the process. They lose the respect and trust of their friends. The most common behaviors of people who hold this stone are backstabbing (cutting people down behind their backs), sarcasm (a word that actually means to tear flesh), and verbal sabotage.

EXERCISE **6.4**

Anger: The Fight Response

He who seeks revenge should dig two graves.
Anonymous

Anger. The word itself brings to mind images of pounding fists, yelling, and smoke pouring out of one's ears and nose. But anger is as natural a human emotion as love. It is universal among all humans. Anger is a survival emotion; it's the fight component of the fight-or-flight response. We use anger to communicate our feelings, from impatience to rage. We employ anger to communicate boundaries and defend values. Studies show that the average person has fourteen to fifteen anger episodes a day. These often arise when our expectations are not met upon demand. Although feeling angry is within the normal limits of human emotions, anger is often mismanaged and misdirected. Unfortunately, we have been socialized to suppress our feelings of anger. As a result, anger either tears us apart from the inside (ulcers) or promotes intermittent eruptions of verbal or physical violence. In most—if not all—cases, we do not deal with our anger correctly.

Research has shown that there are four distinct ways in which people mismanage their anger:

1. **Somatizers:** People who never show any signs of anger and internalize their feelings until eventually there is major bodily damage (e.g., ulcers, temporomandibular joint dysfunction, colitis, or migraines).

2. **Self-punishers:** People who neither repress their anger nor explode, but rather deny themselves a proper outlet for anger because of guilty feelings (e.g., eating, shopping).

3. **Exploders:** Individuals who erupt like a volcano and spread their temper like hot lava, destroying anyone and anything in their path with either verbal or physical abuse.

4. **Underhanders:** Individuals who sabotage others or seek revenge through somewhat socially acceptable behavior (e.g., sarcasm, appearing late for meetings).

Although we tend to employ all of these styles at one time or another, given the situation and prevailing circumstances, we tend to rely on one dominant style of mismanaged anger. What is your most dominant style? What situations provoke an anger response in you? How do you deal with these feelings of anger?

There are some ways to deal with anger correctly or perhaps even creatively. For example, (1) take a time-out from the situation, followed by a time-in to resolve the issue, (2) communicate your feelings diplomatically, (3) learn to think through your anger, (4) plan several options to a situation, (5) lower personal expectations, and, most important, (6) learn to forgive—make past anger pass. What are some ways you can vent your anger creatively?

Although anger is an emotion we all experience and should recognize when it arises, it is crucial to manage it correctly. Sometimes just writing down on paper what gets you frustrated can be the beginning of the resolution process. And anger must be fully resolved.

EXERCISE **6.5**

The Anger Cycle

Mismanaged Anger Cycle: Picking Up Hot Stones

Metaphorically speaking, anger is like a hot stone: If you pick it up to throw at someone, you will get burned. The mismanaged anger cycle begins with the interpretation of some (internal or external) event (step 1) and progresses clockwise (steps 2 through 5) in an unbroken circle of anger (from frustration to rage) in which angry feelings begin and are perpetuated because they are not resolved. Anger as a hot stone burns! The accompanying diagrams depict two cycles of anger. Which can you most relate to?

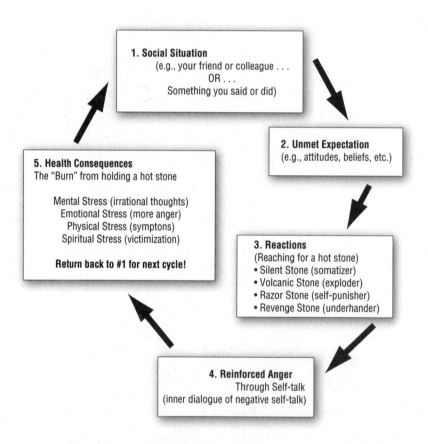

Strategies for Well-Managed Anger: Dropping Hot Stones

In a well-managed anger style, the cycle of anger is broken because the situation and the feelings generated from it are worked through and resolved, starting with step 1 and ending with step 5.

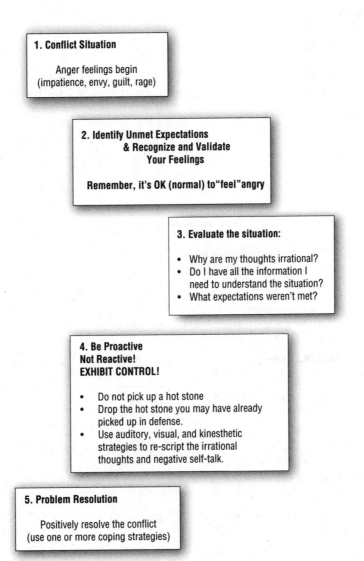

1. Conflict Situation

Anger feelings begin
(impatience, envy, guilt, rage)

**2. Identify Unmet Expectations
& Recognize and Validate
Your Feelings**

Remember, it's OK (normal) to "feel" angry

3. Evaluate the situation:

- Why are my thoughts irrational?
- Do I have all the information I need to understand the situation?
- What expectations weren't met?

**4. Be Proactive
Not Reactive!
EXHIBIT CONTROL!**

- Do not pick up a hot stone
- Drop the hot stone you may have already picked up in defense.
- Use auditory, visual, and kinesthetic strategies to re-script the irrational thoughts and negative self-talk.

5. Problem Resolution

Positively resolve the conflict
(use one or more coping strategies)

EXERCISE **6.6**

Creative Anger Management Skills Action Plan

Dealing with anger effectively means working to resolve the issues and expectations that surface from the anger episode. There are many ways to creatively resolve anger so that you reclaim your emotional sovereignty. The following list is a synthesis of suggestions from a variety of sources. Read through each suggestion, and below it write a description of what steps you can implement to creatively manage your anger and keep each episode of anger within a healthy time period.

1. **Know your anger style.** What is your most predominant mismanaged anger style?

    Somatizer → maybe underhandler?

2. **Learn to self-monitor your anger.** Reflect on the past day's events (including listening to the news), and estimate the number of times you felt anger:

    _3_

3. **Learn to de-escalate your anger.** List three ways to let off steam (e.g., leave the room, take a big sigh, count to ten).
    a. _Walk the dogs (when I am home)_
    b. _leave the situation_
    c. _Request obj. 3rd party be present_

4. **Learn to out-think your anger.** Many times anger results from insufficient information. Identify an anger situation and reprocess the information to neutralize your anger feelings:

    Code Nurse being called →

5. **Get comfortable with all your feelings.** Some people have a hard time saying the phrase "I am angry" or "I feel angry." Are you one of them? Please explain.

    No, I recognize I am angry - just don't always identify the reason effectively

6. **Plan in advance.** Although avoidance is not advocated, making plans to work around a problem is known as the path of least resistance. Identify a current frustration, and then list three things you can do as an action plan to rise above the occasion.
    a. _make a list - stay on task discussion_
    b. _write a response to question that will be asked - & emotional answer_
    c. _____

7. **Develop a strong support system.** List three friends to whom you can turn to vent your frustrations as well as ask to provide an objective opinion about your stressful situation.

   a. _Ruth_

   b. _Elizabeth W._

   c. _Amanda y._

8. **Develop realistic expectations for yourself and others.** Pick one anger situation you have had today (or yesterday), identify the expectation that wasn't met, and then refine the expectation.

   Unmet expectation: _Ø response from meeting request e CHN_

   Refined expectation: _Conciously allow time for a response_

9. **Turn complaints into requests.** As the expression goes, you get more flies with honey than vinegar. Script a phrase that you can use to incorporate the magic of request:

   "_I may have mis-understood, could you tell me again ..._"

10. **Make past anger pass.** Letting go of anger begins with forgiveness. List three people who you feel have violated you in some way and with whom the steps of forgiveness need to be taken to bring closure to the situation.

    a. _Joanie / Joan_

    b. _Tina_

    c. _Marti_

EXERCISE **6.7**

Fear This!

We have nothing to fear but fear itself.
Franklin Delano Roosevelt

Those immortal words, spoken by Roosevelt during the Great Depression, were crafted to calm an unsettled American public. Fear, like anger, is a very normal human emotion. We all experience it—more often than not, too many times in the course of our lives. Fear tends to be a difficult emotion to resolve. Feelings of anxiety or fear can trickle down from the mind to the body and wreak physical havoc from head to toe. Whereas anger tends to make one want to defend turf and fight, fear makes one want to head for the hills and keep on running. The effects of fear can be exhausting. In fact, the effects *do* exhaust the body to the point of disease, illness, and sometimes death. Avoidance isn't the answer, but it's often the technique used to deal with fear.

Although many situations can promote anxiety, there are really only a handful of basic human fears. They include the following:

- *Fear of failure:* A loss of self-worth through an event or action that promotes feelings of self-rejection

- *Fear of rejection:* A loss of self-worth due to a perceived lack of acceptance from someone whose respect is important to you

- *Fear of the unknown:* A fear based on a lack of confidence or inner faith to act without knowledge of future events or circumstances

- *Fear of dying:* Anxiety produced by the pain, suffering, and uncertainty of death

- *Fear of isolation:* A fear of loneliness (also known as abandonment); uncomfortable feelings of solitude

- *Fear of loss of self-control:* The conflict between the inability to determine factors that are and are not controllable and the feeling of responsibility for total control that produces anxiety

Many of these basic human fears are very closely related and overlap in some instances. Some fears may dominate our way of thinking, whereas others don't relate to our lifestyles. Fear of any kind, however, is very much related to our level of self-esteem. When we are down on ourselves, we are most susceptible to situations or circumstances that we perceive as frightening. Like anger, fears *must* be resolved. Resolution does not include ignoring or avoiding the problem. It is not easy, and it takes work. When pursued properly, resolution is a continual process with many fruitful outcomes.

Sometimes by looking at our stressors, we can associate them with specific fears. The following questions may help you reflect on your current stressors that fall into this category.

1. Does one of the basic human fears tend to dominate your list of stressors? If so, why do you suppose that is the case?

2. How do you usually deal with fear? Are you the type of person who hopes the circumstances surrounding these fears will go away?

3. What are some practical ways that will help you deal with some of these major fears?

_____

_____

_____

_____

_____

_____

_____

_____

_____

_____

_____

_____

_____

_____

_____

_____

_____

_____

EXERCISE **6.8**

Confrontation of a Stressor

It happens to us all the time: Someone or something gets us frustrated, and we literally or figuratively head for the hills, either avoiding the person or thing altogether or ignoring the situation in the hope that it will go away. But when we ignore situations like this, they typically come back to haunt us. In the short run, avoidance looks appealing, even safe. But in the long run, it is bad policy. We avoid confrontation because we want to avoid the emotional pain associated with it, the pain our ego suffers. Handled creatively, diplomatically, and rationally, the pain is minimal, and it often helps our spirits grow. After all, this is what life is all about: achieving our full human potential.

The art of peaceful confrontation involves a strategy of creativity, diplomacy, and grace to ensure that you come out the victor, not the victim. In this sense, confrontation doesn't mean a physical battle but rather a mental, emotional, or spiritual battle. Unlike a physical battle where knights wear armor, this confrontation requires that you set aside the shield of your ego long enough to resolve the fear or anger associated with the stressor. The weapons of this confrontation are self-assertiveness, self-reliance, and faith. There is no malice, spite, or deceit involved. Coping mechanisms that aid the confrontation process include, but are not limited to, the following strategies: communication, information seeking, cognitive reappraisal, social engineering, and values assessment and clarification.

We all encounter stressors from which we tend to run away. Now it is time to gather your internal resources and make a plan to successfully confront your stressors. When you initiate this confrontation plan, you will come out the victor with a positive resolution and a feeling of accomplishment. First, reexamine the list of your top ten stressors. Then, select a major stressor to confront and resolve. Prepare a plan of action, and then carry it out. When you return, write about it: what the stressor was, what your strategy was, how it worked, how you felt about the outcome, and, perhaps most important, what you learned from this experience.

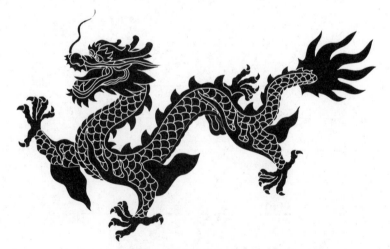

The Stressor

State the stressor you plan to confront here.

_____

_____

_____

_____

_____

_____

Action Plan

State your plan of diplomatic confrontation here.

_____

_____

_____

_____

_____

Emotional Processing

After you have faced your fear, describe here what happened and how you now feel having done this. What did you learn from this experience?

_____

_____

_____

_____

_____

_____

Chapter 6

EXERCISE **6.9**

The Key to Happiness Survey

There are several inventories, questionnaires, and surveys regarding personal happiness. Some are based on momentary happiness (how you feel right now), whereas others are based on happiness as a part of who you are (state vs. trait characteristics). Although some surveys are measured for reliability and validity, by and large happiness is a very subjective state, meaning that you, not a questionnaire, are the only one who can tell if you are really a happy person.

The following questions are based on the ideals of happiness as viewed by the Oxford Happiness Questionnaire and the Authentic Happiness work of Martin Seligman. Although on the actual questionnaires these questions are measured on a scale of 1 to 5, here they are presented as Yes/No statements. Although this survey has not been measured for validity, you can get a pretty good idea of whether happiness is a part of who you are by reading and answering the questions.

1. By and large, I see myself as a happy person.   Yes   No
2. Overall, I am pretty satisfied with the direction of my life.   Yes   No
3. Usually, I wake up excited about the day ahead of me.   Yes   No
4. I tend to surround myself with happy, creative, and confident people.   Yes   No
5. Overall, my level of confidence is rather high with most everything I do.   Yes   No
6. Without a doubt, my life has a meaningful purpose.   Yes   No
7. I take delight in new adventures and discovering life's little surprises.   Yes   No
8. I find myself laughing several times a day, even to myself.   Yes   No
9. When things go badly, I am able to quickly shift my expectations.   Yes   No
10. Even when I am low on money, I can still find exciting things to do.   Yes   No
11. I have very few, if any, regrets about how I have lived my life.   Yes   No
12. I have many positive memories of my life.   Yes   No
13. It's pretty easy to see the good in people and the beauty in things.   Yes   No
14. Overall, I have positive thoughts and feelings about most things.   Yes   No
15. My future is bright and full of potential.   Yes   No
16. I can and do laugh at my own mistakes.   Yes   No
17. I can find time to do the things I really wish to do.   Yes   No
18. Overall, I feel that I have a sense of control/direction in my life.   Yes   No
19. I can be as happy in the company of others as I can be by myself.   Yes   No
20. I have a good amount of physical, mental, and spiritual energy.   Yes   No

Key: As stated earlier, this survey does not have a validated measure. However, if you responded "yes" to over half of the questions, consider yourself to be a happy person. If you responded "no" to over half of these statements, and you would like to have more happiness in your life, ask yourself what steps you can take to shift the perceptions highlighted in this survey to balance your scale of emotions.

Additional thoughts on your level of happiness:

_____

_____

_____

_____

_____

_____

_____

EXERCISE **6.10**

Emotional Well-Being

Emotional well-being is best described as "the ability to feel and express the entire range of human emotions, and to control them, not be controlled by them." Sounds like a pretty tall order, huh? Well, it doesn't have to be.

What is the range of human emotions? Everything from anger to love, and all that's in between. No emotion is excluded, meaning that it is perfectly all right to feel angry, jealous, giddy, sad, depressed, light-hearted, and silly. All of these feelings comprise the total human experience, the complete spectrum of human emotions.

A well-accepted theory suggests that early in our development, we spend the greatest amount of time trying on and exploring emotions. But if you are like most people, you were told at an early age one or more of the following expressions related to your behavior: "Wipe that smile off your face," "Big boys don't cry," "Don't you ever talk back to me," or "I'll give you something to cry about." Perhaps our parents had good intentions, or perhaps they were just at wit's end. Regardless of what prompts such comments, most youngsters interpret the message altogether differently than intended. Instead of relating such phrases only to the moment, most children take the meaning of such messages globally and think it is never all right to laugh or to cry. If we hear these messages enough, we begin to deny some of our feelings by stuffing them down into our unconscious minds—only to meet them head-on later in life.

The second half of the emotional well-being equation says that to be emotionally well, we must control our feelings, not let them control us. Our feelings control us when we refuse to feel and express them or when we linger too long in the moods of anger, anxiety, depression, grief, or boredom. The result is stagnation, not dynamic living.

Here are some questions to ponder about your own sense of emotional well-being:

1. What is your least favorite emotion, one that you don't like to feel or perhaps would rather avoid feeling? Can you explain why?

2. Combing through your memory, can you remember a time (or times) when you were told or reminded not to act or feel a certain way (e.g., big boys don't cry), or were perhaps even humiliated? Take a moment to describe this incident.

3. What is your favorite emotion? Why? How often would you say you feel this emotion throughout the course of a typical day?

4. If you feel you may be the kind of person who doesn't acknowledge or express your emotions, can you think of ways to change your behavior and begin to gain a sense of emotional balance?

_____

_____

_____

Personality Traits

EXERCISE **7.1**

Under the Gun: Stress and Personality

Pick a stressor in your life and explain the characteristics that you feel you employ to deal with stress based on the concepts of the hardy personality.

1. Control: _____

   _____

2. Commitment: _____

   _____

3. Challenge: _____

   _____

List any other aspects (inner resources) that help you get through the tough times:

1. _____

2. _____

3. _____

4. _____

Do you have any attributes in common with the Type A behavior? If so, list them here:

1. _____

2. _____

3. _____

4. _____

When push comes to shove, we all have some survival skills. What biphasic traits do you utilize to survive?

1. _____

2. _____

3. _____

EXERCISE **7.2**

Stress-Prone Personality Survey

The following is a survey based on the traits of the codependent personality. Please answer the following questions with the most appropriate number.

4 = Always   3 = Often   2 = Sometimes   1 = Rarely   0 = Never

1. I tend to seek approval (acceptance) from others (e.g., friends, colleagues, family members).   **④** 3 2 1 0

2. I have very strong perfection tendencies.   4 **③** 2 1 0

3. I am usually involved in many projects at one time.   **④** 3 2 1 0

4. I rise to the occasion in times of crisis.   4 **③** 2 1 0

5. Despite problems with my family, I will always defend them.   4 **③** 2 1 0

6. I have a tendency to put others before myself.   4 **③** 2 1 0

7. I don't feel appreciated for all the things I do.   4 3 **②** 1 0

8. I tend to tell a lot of white lies.   4 3 **②** 1 0

9. I will help most anyone in need.   4 3 **②** 1 0

10. I tend to trust others' perceptions rather than my own.   4 3 **②** 1 0

11. I have a habit of overreacting to situations.   4 **③** 2 1 0

12. Despite great achievements, my self-esteem usually suffers.   4 **③** 2 1 0

13. My family background is better described as victim than victor.   4 **③** 2 1 0

14. I have been known to manipulate others with acts of generosity and favors.   4 3 2 **①** 0

15. I am really good at empathizing with my friends and family.   **④** 3 2 1 0

16. I usually try to make the best impression possible with people.   **④** 3 2 1 0

17. I like to validate my feelings with others' perceptions.   4 **③** 2 1 0

18. I am an extremely well-organized individual.   4 **③** 2 1 0

19. It's easier for me to give love and much more difficult to receive it.   4 **③** 2 1 0

20. I tend to hide my feelings if I know they will upset others.   4 **③** 2 1 0

Total score _____ **58**

Score: A score of more than 30 points indicates that you most likely have traits associated with the codependent personality, a personality style known to be stress-prone.

EXERCISE 7.3

Stress-Resistant Personality Survey

The following survey is composed of statements based on the hardy, survivor, and risk-taking personality traits—all of which share common aspects that resist rather than attract or promote stress in one's life. Please answer the following questions with the most appropriate number.

4 = Always   3 = Often   2 = Sometimes   1 = Rarely   0 = Never

1. I wake up each morning ready to face a new day.	4	3	2	(1)	0
2. I tend not to let fear run my life.	4	3	(2)	1	0
3. I would consider myself to be an optimist.	4	3	(2)	1	0
4. I tend to see "problems" as opportunities for personal growth and success.	4	3	(2)	1	0
5. Although I like to be in control of my fate, I know when to go with the flow when things are out of my control.	4	3	(2)	1	0
6. Curiosity is one of my stronger attributes.	(4)	3	2	1	0
7. Life isn't always fair, but I still manage to enjoy myself.	4	3	(2)	1	0
8. When things knock me off balance, I am resilient and get back on my feet quickly.	4	3	(2)	1	0
9. My friends would say that I have the ability to turn misfortune into luck.	4	3	2	1	(0)
10. I believe that if you don't take risks, you live a boring life and won't get far.	4	3	(2)	1	0
11. I like to think of myself as being a creative person.	4	3	(2)	1	0
12. I believe in the philosophy that "one person truly can make a difference."	4	(3)	2	1	0
13. I am both organized and flexible with my life's day-to-day schedule.	4	(3)	2	1	0
14. Sometimes having nothing to do is the best way to spend a day.	4	3	2	1	(0)
15. I trust that I am part of a greater force of life in the universe.	(4)	3	2	1	0
16. I believe in the philosophy that "you make your own breaks."	4	3	(2)	1	0
17. I approach new situations with the idea that I will learn something valuable, regardless of the outcome.	(4)	3	2	1	0
18. When I start a project, I see it through to its successful completion.	4	(3)	2	1	0
19. I am strong willed, which I see as a positive characteristic to accomplish hard tasks.	4	3	2	1	(0)
20. I am committed to doing my best in most everything in life.	(4)	3	2	1	0

Total score _____44_____

Score: A score of more than 30 points indicates that you most likely have traits associated with the hardy, survivor, and calculated risk-taker personalities, personality types known to be stress-resistant.

EXERCISE **7.4**

Giving Your Self-Esteem a Healthy Boost

Self-esteem is thought to be composed of five aspects: uniqueness, empowerment, role models, connectedness, and calculated risk-taking. With this in mind, let's take a look at your level of self-esteem with respect to these five areas. Try to answer the following questions as best you can.

I: Uniqueness

List five characteristics or personal attributes that make you feel special and unique (e.g., sense of humor, being a good cook, a passion for travel):

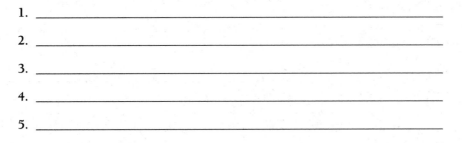

1. _____
2. _____
3. _____
4. _____
5. _____

II: Empowerment

List five areas or aspects of your life in which you feel you are empowered:

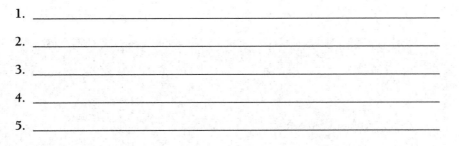

1. _____
2. _____
3. _____
4. _____
5. _____

III: Mentors and Role Models

Name five people (heroes, mentors, or role models) who have one or more characteristics that you admire and wish to emulate or enhance as a part of your own personality. Please describe the person and the trait or traits.

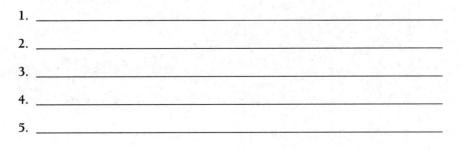

1. _____
2. _____
3. _____
4. _____
5. _____

IV: Social Support Groups

Friends and family are now thought to be crucial to one's health status. To have a sense of belonging is very important in one's life. Who (or what) gives you a sense of belonging? Please describe each in a sentence.

1. _____

2. _____

3. _____

4. _____

5. _____

V: Calculated Risk-Taking

List five good risks that you have taken in the past year that you feel have augmented your sense of self-worth and courage.

1. _____

2. _____

3. _____

4. _____

5. _____

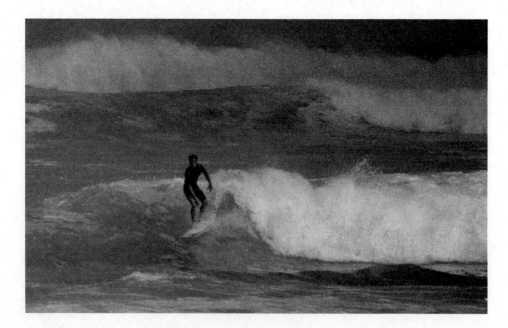

EXERCISE **7.5**

Perfection versus Excellence

Are you a perfectionist? Perhaps at some level we all are. Some people demand quality regarding only a few things about which they are passionate. Others seem to be anal retentive about everything. Everything has to be just perfect: hair, homework, the wax job on the car, the table setting, the volume level of the speakers, or balancing the checkbook to the nearest penny. This is the kind of person who drives you crazy. And if you are one of these people, you probably drive *yourself* crazy. Being driven crazy is another word for stress, and it's no secret that perfectionism and stress go hand in hand, because as hard as you try, nothing will ever be perfect.

For some people, perfectionism is a survival skill. Keeping things neat and tidy means there is less chance of being yelled at by an alcoholic or abusive parent. Whereas there are some who believe that perfectionism is a learned trait, others believe that being a perfectionist is a function of your zodiac sign (Virgos and Pisces are said to be the worst).

Perfection isn't an absolute thing—it's relative, if it even exists at all. The truth is that nothing is perfect. Perfection is merely an illusion, and you will drive yourself crazy if you try to achieve it.

Excellence, unlike perfection, isn't an absolute thing. Although it may sound like a duel of semantics, there *is* a difference between excellence and perfectionism. Excellence is a culmination of desire and talents that brings out the best in every situation while at the same time enjoying the process (eustress) as it unfolds. Perfectionism is a form of neurotic behavior that falls under the domain of obsessive-compulsive behavior. Like an addiction, when the current project is done, satisfaction isn't achieved until the next project is done to perfection. Excellence is a focus of talents and abilities on a few things. Perfectionism is an attitude projected onto everything. Whereas searching for excellence is good, and in many cases is actually encouraged, the drive for perfectionism actually promotes stress.

1. Do you have perfectionistic tendencies? If so, why do you suppose you are like this?

2. How do the concepts of excellence and perfection differ for you? Please explain.

3. List three things in your life in which you strive for excellence, and then briefly explain how you best accomplish this.

4. If you find your perfectionistic habits getting the better of you, what are two things you can do to change or modify these behaviors?

_____

_____

_____

_____

87

EXERCISE **7.6**

Role Models and Heroes

Everything I do and say with anyone makes a difference.
Gita Bellen

It has been said that since the advent of television and video technology, the culture of American heroes has changed significantly, if it has not disappeared altogether. At the turn of the twenty-first century, a popular weekly magazine conducted a survey identifying current American heroes. It showed that the top 25 people selected were either movie stars, television actors, or rock musicians. Today people are still fascinated with celebrities' ideals of fame and fortune. Simply stated, we live in a celebrity culture.

In days gone by there was a different fascination that created legends, catapulted individuals to hero status, and inspired people to follow in their footsteps. The early American heroes and role models were the inventors, the explorers, the philosophers, and the movers and shakers of the world—for example, Ben Franklin, Florence Nightingale, Babe Ruth, Booker T. Washington, Mark Twain, Lewis and Clark, Amelia Earhart, Carl Jung, Abraham Lincoln, Eleanor Roosevelt, Charles Lindbergh, Thomas Edison, Harriet Tubman, Henry David Thoreau, Rosa Parks, John Glenn, and Lance Armstrong.

It's quite well known that we are capable of heroic deeds, and there are a great many unrecognized heroes currently in our midst. These are just ordinary people who do extraordinary things, people who give 100 percent effort against insurmountable odds and come out on top. If you were to ask a child who his or her hero is, you might likely hear the reply "Mom" or "Dad." In the course of a lifetime, however, a great many people influence us; some we never meet but perhaps only hear or read about. Today, people such as Lance Armstrong, Barack Obama, and many Iraq and Afghanistan war veterans are redefining what it means to be a hero.

When you stop to think about it, some people can have a profound positive influence on our lives—perhaps more than we recognize. The following questions are provided as food for thought regarding your role models and life heroes.

1. What person would you say has had the greatest influence on your life? Why?

2. Most people model their adult behavior and even their thoughts and perceptions as a result of a synthesis of several people and the influence they have had. What people do you admire and tend to model some of your thoughts and behaviors on?

3. If you could have lunch with anyone—living or dead—just once, who would you like to break bread with and tap into for an hour, and why?

4. We not only have role models and heroes, but also are role models. We not only absorb the light, but also reflect it. For whom in your life have you been a role model? Who have you touched, inspired, and reflected upon?

_____

_____

EXERCISE **7.7**

Control: A Double-Edged Sword

"God grant me the serenity to accept the things I cannot change, the courage to change the things I can, and the wisdom to know the difference." The Serenity Prayer, by Reinhold Neibuhr, embodies one of the cornerstone principles of the recovery program initiated by Alcoholics Anonymous. Today it is used in nearly all types of recovery programs in which people work to shed their addictive behaviors, both chemical and behavioral.

The unyielding message of the prayer is about control. Control is a paradox. It can be perceived as either good or bad. For this reason, it can be compared to a double-edged sword. To master this tool and not inflict self-damage, one must understand and recognize what one does and does not have control over and have the wisdom to know the difference. Many people use control as a manipulative behavior. Often they try to control others and events because they find these easier to control than their own thoughts and actions. This manipulative behavior can become addictive. Each episode of control is like the next fix—a false inflation of one's self-worth until the next controllable opportunity arrives. The result can be a vicious circle, and it can be a very unhealthy behavior. Conversely, control is also said to be one of three prime characteristics (in conjunction with challenge and commitment) in what psychologists now refer to as the *hardy personality* or *stress-resistant personality*. Unlike manipulative behavior, this perspective focuses on self-control as a function of willpower.

Are you a master swordsman with a strong sense of self-control, or does the action of manipulative behavior metaphorically cut and nick your hands? Do people and events that you seem to have no control over frustrate you? Do you spend a lot of energy against the flow, managing events that you feel only you can do well? Do you mistake or have you mistaken responsibility for control? How is your sense of willpower? And finally, what are some ways you can become a master swordsman with the power of self-control?

_____

_____

_____

_____

_____

_____

_____

EXERCISE **7.8**

Victimhood

Once a victim, twice a volunteer.
Anonymous

The headlines read: Woman sues fast-food chain because coffee is too hot. Man sues airline for missing flight to wedding. Lawyer of defendant sues lawyer of plaintiff. Perhaps it's no surprise that the United States has more lawyers per capita than any other country in the world. We live in a litigious society in which blame is constantly placed on somebody else and lawsuits are common. Everyone is suing everyone else. Victim consciousness has run rampant in the entitlement generation. Psychologists have another name for this phenomenon: victimhood.

It is easy to blame someone else when things don't go our way. When expectations go unmet, whether it is coffee that burns our tongue or a delayed airline flight, we can easily feel violated. If left unchecked, these feelings of violation can quickly turn to victimization, and revenge seems to be the only solution. The greater the emotional damage, the greater the penalty we wish to inflict on those who we feel have wronged us.

It is fair to say that victimhood in America is at an all-time high, as citizens repeatedly experience unmet expectations. A general feeling of frustration is the precursor to victimhood. At some point, though, we need to realize that we are not passive victims in the game of life. We have an active role in every situation we encounter. There are some things we can control, and there are many we cannot. As the Serenity Prayer suggests, it is wise to know the difference. Moreover, we need to learn to take responsibility, not only for our actions, but also for our feelings.

Is there something you have felt victimized about lately? Grades, term papers, flat tires, or delayed flights? If you have, you're not alone. But take a moment to look at whatever makes you feel victimized right now. Describe the situation as you see it, as you experienced it. Then try to describe it as objectively as possible. Feelings of victimization are often associated with feelings of anger. Can you recognize any feelings of anger when you sense a moment of victimization? Why do you suppose this is so? Knowing the relationship between anger and victimization, can you begin to outline ways in which you can work toward resolving these feelings and perhaps toward acknowledging a greater responsibility for those events in your life, including acceptance of those things you cannot change?

_____

_____

_____

_____

_____

EXERCISE **7.9**

Boosting Your Self-Esteem

Many themes in this workbook revolve around the concept of self-esteem. Self-esteem is considered by many to be the bottom line with regard to perceptions of stressors and, indeed, how we manage our stress. *Self-esteem* is often defined as our level of self-approval. It is used synonymously with *self-worth*, *self-respect*, and *self-value*. Ultimately, strong self-esteem equates to the degree of acceptance and love we bestow upon ourselves. High self-esteem can *sometimes* be mistaken and confused with over-confidence, cockiness, and aggressiveness. So, in a humble effort, we tend to compensate. The result is often modesty to the point of negativism, and negativism perpetuates low self-esteem. Today, society gives many mixed messages that value both humbleness and greatness. The ideal is a fine line that we must learn to walk in balance.

Self-esteem is a complex concept. It includes, but is not limited to, acceptance, love, forgiveness, self-understanding, a personal value system, and atonement. Self-esteem is as hard to measure as it is to define. Suffice it to say that at some level each of us knows generally where our self-esteem is, as well as its daily fluctuations and things that inflate or deflate it. Almost everything we say, think, feel, and do is a function of our self-esteem. In turn, messages that we communicate to ourselves and others from our thoughts, feelings, and actions can reinforce either low or high self-esteem. When our self-esteem is low, we become more susceptible to life's pressures, like a bull's-eye target. Conversely, when we are feeling good about ourselves, problems tend to roll off our backs quite easily. Stress becomes manageable, if it's even recognized. Several factors contribute to strong self-esteem.

- *Uniqueness:* Characteristics that make you feel special
- *Power:* Feelings of self-reliance and self-efficacy
- *Modeling:* Having a mentor or role model to identify with as a guide on your life journey
- *Connectedness:* Feelings of bonding and belonging with others; your network of friends and support groups
- *Calculated risks:* Surveying the odds of your chances of success, then taking the next step if these odds are in your favor

Take a moment to contemplate the idea of self-esteem, what your threshold is, and the bounds in which it oscillates. What are some ways to increase your threshold for a higher level of self-esteem? Do you see a relationship between your current self-esteem threshold and how well you deal with stress? Try to identify five characteristics that make you unique and give you a sense of empowerment, five role models, and five friends or groups of people you consider part of your support system.

_____

_____

EXERCISE **7.10**

I Have No Secrets!

Secrets are the cornerstone of psychological dysfunction.
Gail S., recovering alcoholic

Everybody has a secret or two. There are things in our past that we really don't wish to share with the world. Typically, the things we keep secret are things that make us look bad. Relatives in prison, alcoholic parents, sexual abuse, and drug addictions are just a few of the more common skeletons in the closet, but there are hundreds more.

Here's the problem with secrets: They lead to emotional dysfunction. We try so hard to shove these bones to the back of the closet that they come back to haunt us. Addictions are the prime example of dysfunctional secrets.

Health experts agree that keeping secrets like this is anything but healthy. Having said that, you should know that there is a big difference between secrets and surprises. Secrets are typically things we are ashamed of and try to hide. Surprises are things we tend to hold back on until the appropriate time to acknowledge them. Examples of surprises include presents, engagements, pregnancies, and promotions.

The explanation of the difference between secrets and surprises may be a futile exercise in semantics, but the real message here is not to have any secrets within yourself. To do this, you must be absolutely honest about yourself with yourself. So take some time to comb your mind and ask yourself whether you are keeping any secrets that are causing some level of dysfunction in your life. Are there some skeletons that need to be cremated?

Now is the time to do some cleaning of the closets. To keep a degree of security when you write about your secrets, feel free to use the third person so that you have the freedom to reveal the truth without feeling overexposed. Good luck!

_____

_____

_____

_____

_____

_____

_____

_____

_____

EXERCISE **7.11**

My Locus of Control

The more you depend on forces outside yourself the more you are dominated by them.
Harold Sherman

Several decades ago a psychologist named Julian Rotter presented the idea that there are two human drives—internal and external motivation. Rotter called them internal and external locus of control.

People who have an external locus of control tend to feel that their lives are controlled by outside factors such as the weather, the stars, the government, destiny, and events beyond their own domain. Someone with an external locus of control places blame (or credit) on others for his or her misfortunes (or blessings). People in this category more likely than not see themselves as passive participants in life.

An internal locus of control signifies a vantage point from which an individual sees responsibility as lying within himself or herself. He or she relies on inner strengths and resources. When faced with a problem or difficult situation, people with an internal locus of control stand up to adversity by themselves. They see themselves as having an active, not passive, role in their lives.

Most likely there are few people who epitomize either end of the spectrum, but we tend to gravitate toward one side or the other. In terms of health, a person with an external locus of control would blame a cold, headache, ulcer, or heart attack on somebody or something. Conversely, a person with an internal locus of control would assume responsibility for his or her health. As long as there is no undue guilt associated with it, this is something health care professionals teach daily.

If you were to venture a guess, where would you see yourself on this continuum? Would you most likely see yourself with an internal locus of control or an external locus of control? Perhaps another way to word it is this: Are you easily motivated by trophies, medals, and horoscopes, or does your source of inspiration come primarily from within? Take a few minutes to ponder the concept of health-related locus of control and share your thoughts here.

_____

_____

_____

_____

_____

_____

_____

Stress and Human Spirituality

EXERCISE **8.1**

Stress and Human Spirituality

It may seem as though stress is the absence of human spirituality, but where there is stress, there is a lesson for enhancing the soul-growth process. Take a moment to make a list of your top ten stressors. If you have less than ten, that's fine. If you have more than ten, simply list the top ten concerns, issues, or problems that are on your mind at this time. When you get done, place a check mark next to each stressor that involves issues concerning yourself or other people. Next, place a check mark next to all stressors that involve values or value conflicts (e.g., time, money, privacy, education). Finally, place a check mark next to all stressors that involve or are related to a meaningful purpose in life (e.g., family, education, career, retirement). It is fine to have a stressor with more than one check mark. We'll come back to this theme in upcoming exercises.

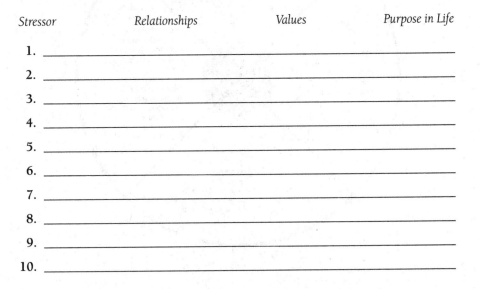

Stressor	Relationships	Values	Purpose in Life
1. _____			
2. _____			
3. _____			
4. _____			
5. _____			
6. _____			
7. _____			
8. _____			
9. _____			
10. _____			

EXERCISE **8.2**

Mandala of the Human Spirit

A *mandala* is a circular-shaped object symbolizing unity, with four separate quarters that represent directions of the universe, seasons of the years, or four points of reference. The mandala can be traced to the dawn of humankind. Mandalas vary in size, design, colors, and symbolism. They are often used in meditation as a focal point of concentration. In addition, they are used as decorations in many cultures, from the Native American medicine wheel to depictions in art from the Far East.

The mandala of the human spirit is a symbol of wholeness. It is a tool of self-awareness to allow you the opportunity to reflect on some of the components of the human spirit: a meaningful purpose in your life, personal values, and the implicit chance to learn more about yourself in precious moments of solitude. Each quadrant represents a direction of your life, with a symbol of orientation. The east is the point of origin. It represents the rising sun, the point of origin for each day. The focus of the mandala then moves southward, then to the west, and finally to the north.

Each focal point of the mandala of the human spirit provides questions for reflection. Take a few moments to reflect on the directions of the mandala to get a better perspective on the well-being of your human spirit. Then draw a circle, divide it into four areas, and fill in the answers to the respective questions, creating a mandala of your very own human spirit (see next page for blank mandala).

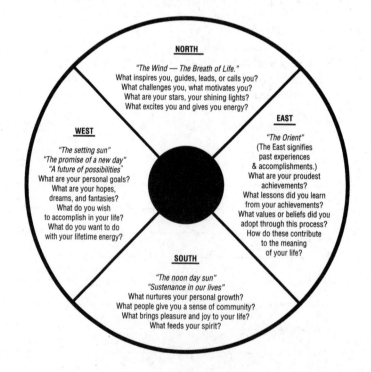

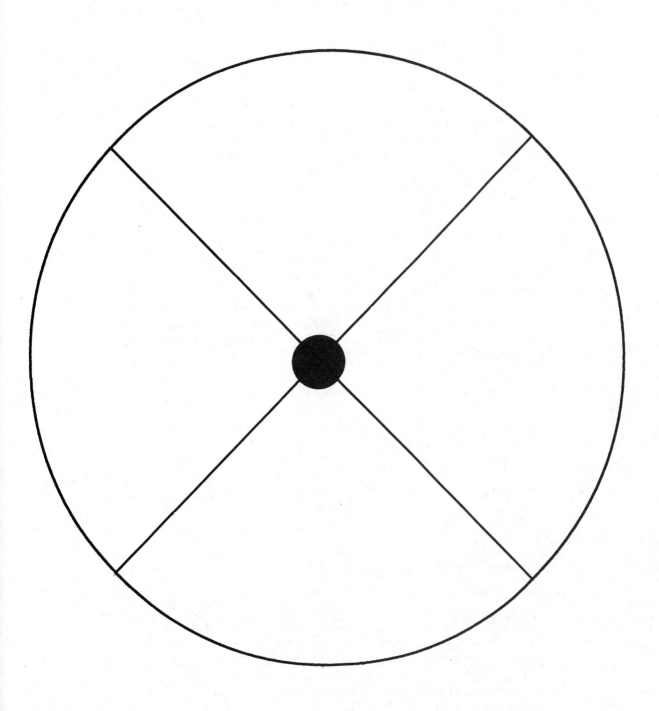

EXERCISE **8.3**

The Three Pillars of Human Spirituality

Every crisis over the age of 30 is a spiritual crisis. Spiritual crises require spiritual cures.
Carl Gustav Jung

The shamans, healers, sages, and wisdom keepers of all times, all continents, and all peoples, in their ageless wisdom, say that human spirituality is composed of three aspects: relationships, values, and purpose in life. These three components are so tightly integrated that it may be hard to separate them from each other. But if this were possible, take a moment to reflect on each aspect of human spirituality to determine the status of your spiritual well-being.

I. Relationships

All life is relationship. In simple terms, there are two categories of relationships: internal (your domestic policy)—how you deal with yourself, how you nurture the relationship with yourself and your higher self—and external (your foreign policy)—how you relate, support, and interact with those people (and all living entities) in your environment. How would you evaluate your internal relationship and what steps could you take to cultivate it? Moving from the aspect of domestic policy to foreign policy, how would you evaluate your external relationships?

_____

_____

_____

_____

_____

II. Your Personal Value System

We each have a value system composed of core and supporting values. Core values (about four to six) are those that form the foundation of our personal belief system. Supporting values support the core values. Intangible core values (e.g., love, honesty, freedom) and supporting values (e.g., education, creativity, and integrity) are often symbolized in material possessions. Quite regularly, our personal value system tends to go through a reorganization process, particularly when there are conflicts in our values. What are your core and supporting values? Please list them in the space provided.

Core Values	*Supporting Values*
1. _____	1. _____
2. _____	2. _____
3. _____	3. _____
4. _____	4. _____
5. _____	5. _____

III. A Meaningful Purpose in Life

A meaningful purpose in life is that which gives our life meaning. Some might call it a life mission. Although it is true that we may have an overall life mission, it is also true that our lives are a collection of meaningful purposes. Suffering awaits those times in between each purpose. What would you say is your life mission, and what purpose are you now supporting to accomplish this mission?

_____

_____

_____

_____

_____

_____

_____

_____

_____

_____

_____

_____

EXERCISE **8.4**

Personal and Interpersonal Relationships

It is often said that all life is relationship—how we deal with ourselves and how we relate to everything else in our lives. It's no secret that relationships can cause stress. For this reason alone, all relationships need nurturing to some degree. Reflect for a moment on all the many relationships that you hold in your life, including the most important relationship—that which you hold with yourself. Relationships also constitute the foundation of your support system.

Relationships go further than friends and family. This core pillar of human spirituality includes our relationship with the air we breathe, the water we drink, and the ground on which we walk. How is your relationship with your environment? Write your name in the center circle and then begin to fill in the circles with the names of those people, places, and things that constitute your relationship with life. Finally, place an asterisk (*) next to those relationships that need special nurturing and then make a strategy by which to start this process.

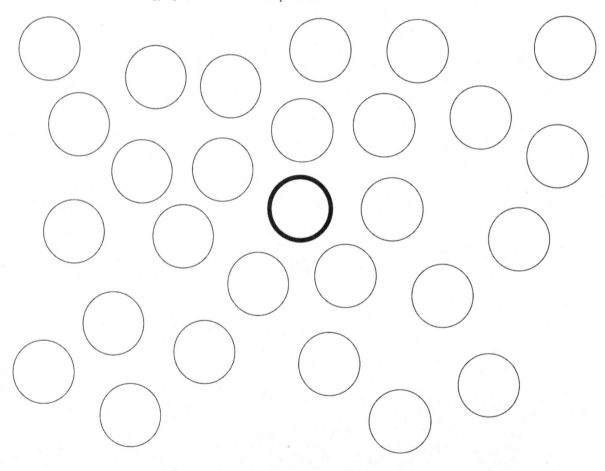

EXERCISE **8.5**

Your Personal Value System

We all have a personal value system—a core pillar of the human spirit that is constantly undergoing renovation. What does your value system currently look like? Perhaps this diagram can give you some insights and, in turn, help resolve some issues that might be causing stress.

The circle in the center represents your core values: abstract or intangible constructs of importance that can be symbolized by a host of material possessions. It is believed that we hold about four to six core values that constitute our personal belief system, which, like a compass, guide the spirit on our human journey. Give this concept some thought and then write in this circle what you consider to be your current core values (e.g., love, happiness, health).

The many circles that surround the main circle represent your supporting values: those values that lend support to your core values (these typically number from five to twelve). Take a moment to reflect on what these might be and then assign one value per small circle. Inside each small circle, include what typically symbolizes that value for you (e.g., wealth can be symbolized by money, a car, or a house). Finally, consider whether any stress you feel in your life is the result of a conflict between your supporting and core values.

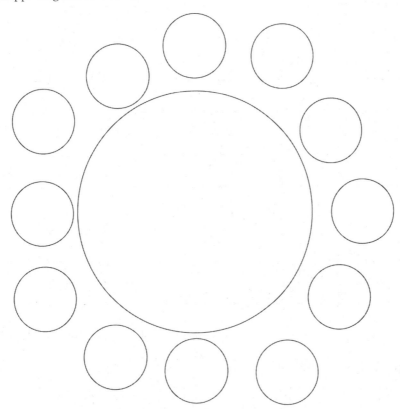

EXERCISE **8.6**

Your Meaningful Purpose in Life

Knowing that your purpose in life may change many times in the course of your life, for this exercise, first write down (in a few words to a sentence) what you consider to be your life purpose now, at this point in time. Then take a moment to briefly describe what you considered to be your purpose in life at the start of each decade of your life (e.g., at age 20 it might be or have been to graduate with a college degree; at age 30 it might be or have been to raise a family or start a business).

Now _____

_____

Age 60 _____

_____

Age 50 _____

_____

Age 40 _____

_____

Age 30 _____

_____

Age 20 _____

_____

Age 16 _____

_____

EXERCISE **8.7**

Roadblocks on the Human Path

If our experience on the human path is, indeed, the evolution of our soul-growth process, then roadblocks can metaphorically be used to describe a temporary halt to this evolutionary process. Roadblocks on the human path are not necessarily aspects in our lives that separate us from our divine source or mission—even though they may seem like this at times. Rather, roadblocks are part of the human path. And although they may initially seem to stifle or inhibit our spiritual growth, this only occurs if we give up or give in to them and do nothing. In the words of a Nazi concentration camp survivor, "Giving up is a final solution to a temporary problem."

Roadblocks take many forms, including unresolved anger or fear, greed, apathy, laziness, excessive judgment, and denial, just to name a few. More often than not, these obstacles manifest symbolically as problems, issues, and concerns (and sometimes people). Although the first thing we may want to do when coming upon a road-block is retreat and do an about-face, avoidance only serves to postpone the inevitable. Miles down the road, we will encounter the same obstacles. Roadblocks must be dealt with.

First make a list of what you consider to be some of the major (tangible) obstacles on your human journey (e.g., the boss from hell, the ex-spouse from hell). Take a moment to identify each with a sentence or two.

1. _____

2. _____

3. _____

4. _____

5. _____

Next, identify what emotions are associated with each roadblock just listed. What emotions do they elicit, and why do you suppose these emotions surface for you as these obstacles come into view?

1. _____

2. _____

3. _____

4. _____

5. _____

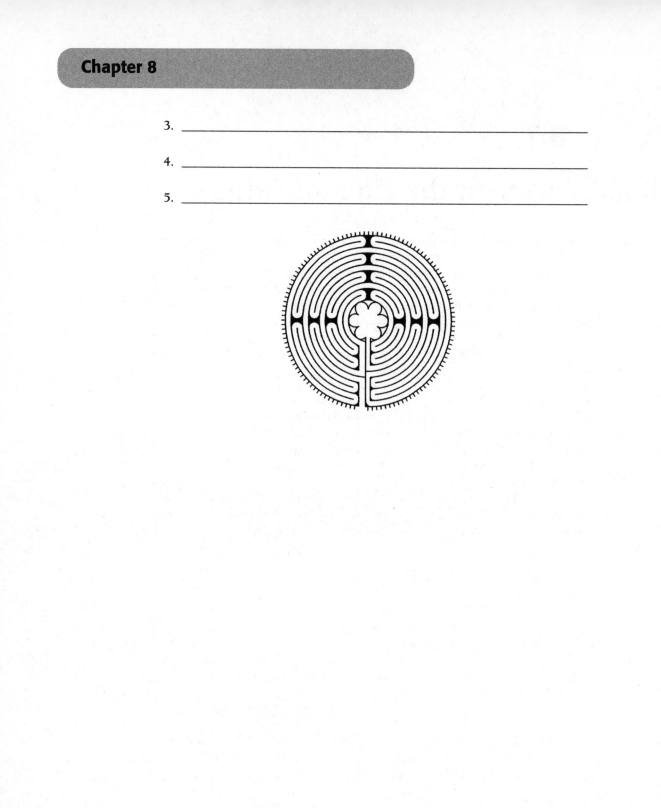

EXERCISE **8.8**

Distractions on the Human Path

Distractions can best be described as those things that pull us off the spiritual path indefinitely. Distractions begin as attractions, but their allure can often cast a spell of slumber on the soul-growth process. Although a respite on the human journey is desirable, and even necessary at times, a prolonged distraction will ultimately weaken our spiritual resolve. The human spirit, like energy, must flow, never stagnate.

The lessons of distractions are quite common in fairy tales. Whether it is the story of Pinocchio or Hansel and Gretel, the warnings regarding distractions are as plentiful as the distractions themselves. The lessons of distractions are common in the great spiritual teachings as well. Here they are called *temptations*. Not always, but often, attractions that become distractions have an addictive quality to them.

What happens when we become distracted? Metaphorically speaking, we fall asleep on the human path. Like Dorothy and her friends on the way to Oz who stepped off the yellow brick road to smell the poppies and fell fast asleep, we too lose our direction, our mission, and our energy stagnates. The end result is never promising.

Unlike roadblocks, distractions are not meant to be circumvented, dismantled, or even transcended. Rather, they are meant to be appreciated—perhaps from afar, perhaps enjoyed briefly and then left behind. Fairy tales aside, what are contemporary distractions? Common examples of everyday distractions might include social contacts, alcohol, television, cell phones, and the Internet.

Take a moment to reflect on what might be some distractions in your life. Make a list and describe each one in a sentence or two. Upon recognition of these, what steps can you take to wake up and get back on the path?

1. _____

   _____

2. _____

   _____

3. _____

   _____

4. _____

   _____

5. _____

   _____

EXERCISE **8.9**

On Being a Good Mystic

In a recent Harris poll, over 70 percent of those questioned admitted to having a mystical experience. It's likely the number is even higher. There are many types of mystical experiences, many of which defy description, but by not attempting to articulate them into a comprehensible language, we begin to forget details of fragments that initially lingered in the mind. By writing them down we make the intangible slightly more tangible, the supernatural a little more natural, and the ordinary a little more extraordinary.

1. Beyond the five senses: What experiences have you had that you consider to be of a mystical, divine nature? Please take a moment to describe two or three of the most memorable ones here.

   _____

   _____

   _____

   _____

2. Renowned psychologist Carl Jung spent the better part of his professional career exploring the mystical nature of the mind. Much of his research involved dreams and dream analysis. He was of the opinion that not only are we capable of precognitive dreams and premonitions, but also that these are common occurrences. Do you recall any dreams that foretold future events? Please explain them here.

   _____

   _____

   _____

   _____

3. The word *synchronicity* was coined by Carl Jung as a means to describe two seemingly random events that come together with great significance. More than just a coincidence, synchronistic events are often thought to be divine messages, when we take the time to decode them. As the expression goes, "There is no such thing as a coincidence. It's God's way of remaining anonymous." What unusual coincidences have you had that are worth noting?

   _____

   _____

   _____

   _____

4. Abraham Maslow coined the phrase "peak experience" to convey a sense of oneness with the universe. People who experience this sensation describe it as "touching the face of God." Although these experiences are often beyond description, describe as best you can in words, through metaphor, simile, or analogy, what this experience was like.

_____

_____

_____

_____

5. To be a good mystic means to appreciate the mystery of life. M. Scott Peck, author of the acclaimed book _The Road Less Traveled_, stated that the highest stage of spiritual growth was to explore the mystery of life but never lose one's appreciation for it. To some, the mystical side of life—those things that cannot be explained rationally through the framework of Western science—is baffling. It leads to a sense of frustration rather than a sense of appreciation. Where do you fall on this continuum?

_____

_____

_____

_____

_____

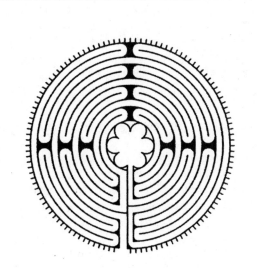

EXERCISE **8.10**

Seasons of the Soul

The planet Earth passes through four distinct seasons as it travels around the sun. As we travel on the human journey, we too pass through many seasonal changes. If you were to talk to the shamans, healers, sages, mystics, and wisdom keepers of all times and ages, you would learn that the human soul has four distinct seasons as well, very similar in nature to the seasons of the earth. These seasons are known by many different names, but the cyclical process is universal in both scope and style. These are the seasons of the soul:

- **The centering process (autumn):** A time to go within and focus on the self. It is a time of soul-searching, a time of self-reflection during which one quiets the mind to calm the soul. It is a time to be still. The centering process is a time to "enter the heart."

- **The emptying process (winter):** A time to release, let go, and detach from thoughts, attitudes, beliefs, and perceptions that at one time may have served us but now only seem to hold us back. For some, this season (known as the void) becomes the dark night of the soul. Sadly, this season is where most people get stuck. It's also known as the "winter of discontent." This is the one season people tend to avoid and, as a consequence, get stuck in. The emptying process is not a pit of despair; it is the womb of creation. But we must take that first step.

- **The grounding process (spring):** A time to seek and process the answers to life's problems and challenges. Sometimes we must wait for an insight; however, the grounding process is augmented by cultivating the silence of the mind. Remember, Nature abhors a vacuum. By making space in the emptying process, new insights or wisdom will make itself known to you. When the pupil is ready, the teacher will come. The grounding process is time to access our intuition and perhaps even attain a feeling of enlightenment in preparation for the next stage (season) of our life journey. This insight, this nugget of wisdom, is the vision of the vision quest.

- **The connecting process (summer):** A season when we come back "home" to our community and share what we have learned from our most recent experience and the wisdom gained from the grounding process. (Remember, greed is not a spiritual value.) The connecting process is based on the premise of love—nurturing our connections with friends, family, and acquaintances (even strangers). As such, the connecting process is a time of celebration. Careful, though—many people tend to get stuck here too.

What makes life challenging, if not difficult at times, is that we are simultaneously experiencing different seasons in regard to different life aspects (problems). For instance, we may be in the emptying process in one aspect of our lives (e.g., career) while smack in the middle of the connecting process for another (e.g., a daughter's wedding). Matters become more complex when a loved one (e.g., spouse) experiencing the same situation (e.g., the death of a child) is in one season while we are in another.

EXERCISE **8.11**

Your Seasons of the Soul

Centering, emptying, grounding, and connecting constitute the four seasons of the soul. Now is the time to take stock of your life. Are you in the midst of one particular season at the present time? Like the planet Earth, we can have many seasons occurring at the same time. There is a normal procession of these seasons; however, it is easy to get stuck in one particular season of the soul. The emptying process is one season most people try to avoid, only to remain stuck there the longest.

Based on the concepts explained in this chapter, take a moment to identify where you feel you are at this time in your life. Please identify what you normally do in each season to get the most out of it. Is there a season you choose to skip? If so, why? Do you take periodic time to do some quality soul-searching? Of these four seasons, is there one that seems to hold the most importance for you? If so, why? How would you describe your connecting process?

The Centering Process (Autumn)

_____

_____

_____

_____

_____

_____

The Emptying Process (Winter)

_____

_____

_____

_____

_____

_____

The Grounding Process (Spring)

_____

_____

_____

_____

_____

_____

The Connecting Process (Summer)

_____

_____

_____

_____

_____

_____

Additional Thoughts

Does the concept of the seasons of the soul help you put your major stressors in perspective? If so, please explain. Please add any additional thoughts here as well.

_____

_____

_____

_____

_____

_____

_____

_____

_____

EXERCISE **8.12**

Muscles of the Soul

Giving up is the final solution to a temporary problem.
Gerta Weizt, Nazi concentration camp survivor

Just as a circle is a universal symbol of wholeness, so too is the butterfly. Given the fact that butterflies, unlike the lowly caterpillar, have wings to fly, butterflies are also considered a symbol of transformation. They can rise above what was once considered a limiting existence. There is a story of a boy who, upon seeing a young butterfly trying to emerge from its chrysalis, tried to help by pulling apart the paper cocoon that housed the metamorphosis. The boy's mother, who saw what he was about to do, quickly stopped him by explaining that the butterfly strengthens its young wings by pushing through the walls of the cocoon. In doing so, its wings become strong enough to fly.

If you were to talk with people who have emerged gracefully from a difficult situation, they would most likely tell you that the muscles they used to break through their barrier(s) included patience, humor, forgiveness, optimism, humbleness, creativity, persistence, courage, willpower, and love. Some people call these traits *inner resources*. I call them "muscles of the soul." These are the muscles we use to dismantle, circumnavigate, and transcend the roadblocks and obstacles in life. Like physical muscles, these muscles will never disappear; however, they will atrophy with disuse. We are given ample opportunity to exercise these muscles, yet not everyone does.

Using the butterfly illustration, write in the wings those attributes, inner resources, and muscles of the soul that you feel help you get through the tough times with grace and dignity, rather than feeling victimized. If there are traits you wish to include to augment the health of your human spirit, yet you feel aren't quite there, write those outside the wings and then draw an arrow into the wings, giving your soul a message that you wish to include (strengthen) these as well. Finally, if you have a box of crayons or pastels, color in your butterfly. Then hang it up on the fridge or bathroom mirror—some place where you can see it regularly—to remind yourself of your spiritual health and your innate ability to transcend life's problems, big and small.

Exercising Your Muscles of the Soul

In his study of several hundred remarkable people, renowned psychologist Abraham Maslow searched for personality traits that culminated in what he called the "self-actualized" person: an individual who was able to rise above the stressors of everyday life and reach his or her highest human potential. In recent years, the term "hardy personality" has been used to explain those people who deal with life's changes in the ever-changing workforce. Researchers Maddi and Kobasa reduced Maslow's self-actualization to three traits: challenge, control, and commitment. In my own research, I have found that there are several more traits than those three which allow one to stand tall, yet go with the flow, particularly after experiencing a life-threatening event that can best be described as "a trip to hell and back."

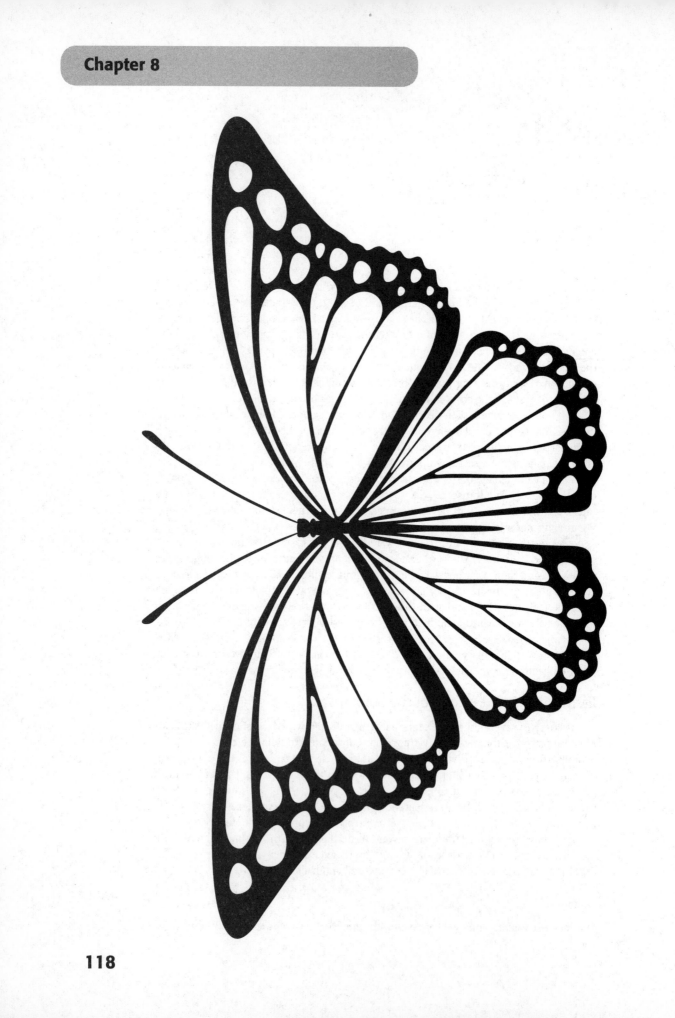

There are two ways to emerge from a proverbial trip to hell. The first is as a victim, where one carries a sense of remorse or resentment for a very long time—sometimes forever. The second is as a victor, an individual who emerges gracefully with neither animosity nor resentment. These people shine! In doing so, they serve as role models for the rest of us. In my research to understand just how these people emerged gracefully, I discovered that they describe a collection of inner resources that I have now come to call "muscles of the soul." More often than not, people use many of these together; however, one muscle seems to shine above the rest. The following list provides a brief highlight of several muscles of the soul.

- **Compassion.** To love without reciprocation, to care for someone or something without recognition or reward—this is compassion. Compassion is the ability to feel and express love when fear is an easier choice. Mother Teresa was compassion personified. You don't have to be a saint to feel compassion. Love is the fabric of our soul.

- **Courage.** The word *courage* comes to the English language via two French words meaning *big heart*. Courage often brings to mind the idea of bravery, and this is certainly a hallmark of courage. Perhaps courage is best thought of as the opposite of fear, for it is courage that allows one to go forward, whereas fear holds one back. Courage is a brave heart.

- **Creativity.** Creativity is two parts imagination, one part organization, one part inspiration, and one part perspiration. Creativity is not a right-brain function; it is an inner resource that requires both hemispheres of the brain. Creativity starts with imagination and then makes the ideas happen. Creativity is the synthesis of imagination and ingenuity.

- **Curiosity.** In the effort to learn, the soul has a wide streak of curiosity. Some may call this an inquiring mind, whereas others call it information seeking. Either way, seeking options, answers, and ideas to learn makes life's journey more interesting.

- **Faith.** Faith is one part optimism, one part love, and two parts mystery. Faith is more than a belief that things will work out OK; it is an innate certainty that all will end well. Faith is an inherent knowledge that we are part of a much bigger whole and that the whole has a loving, divine nature to it.

- **Forgiveness.** Forgiveness is the capacity to pardon those who we feel have violated us, as well as the capacity to forgive ourselves for our mistakes and foibles. Forgiveness is not letting someone off the hook when we feel violated or victimized; rather, it is a gift of compassion we give ourselves so that we can move on. If someone else benefits, great, but forgiveness isn't done for someone else. It is done for ourselves. We must learn to forgive ourselves as well.

- **Humbleness.** The ego begs to go first. The soul is content going last. Humbleness is a trait that is called upon when we are reminded to serve others. Humbleness is manifested in acts of politeness, yet it never undermines self-esteem. Humbleness is based on the Golden Rule, namely, that you should treat others as you would have them treat you. In a fast-paced world where rudeness prevails, acts of humbleness are greatly appreciated.

- **Humor.** Humor is a mental perception that makes us giggle and laugh. Humor isn't a mood, but it can promote a positive mood of happiness. Between parody and irony, between double entendres and slapstick humor, there are literally hundreds of things to make our lips curl and faces laugh. Mark Twain once said that humor is mankind's greatest blessing. There are many people who insist that a sense of humor is what truly saved their lives in times of stress.

- **Integrity.** When you meet someone of integrity, the first thought that comes to mind is honesty. Although this is certainly the cornerstone of integrity, there is more. Integrity is honesty over time. It is a code of conduct with a pledge to the highest ideals in the lowest of times. Integrity literally means the integration of many muscles of the soul.

- **Intuition.** This muscle of the soul may not help you win lottery tickets, but it is useful in sensing good from bad, right from wrong, and up from down. Research delving into the lateralization of the brain into left and right hemispheres suggests that intuition is a right-brain function. Intuition is an inherent knowing about something before the ego jumps in to confuse things. Premonitions, sudden insights, intuitive thoughts, inspiration, and pure enlightenment are examples of how this level of consciousness surfaces in everyday use.

- **Optimism.** Optimism is an inherent quality of being positive. This is not to say that every stressor is meant to be treated as a Pollyanna moment. Rather, optimism is seeing the best in a bad situation. A great definition of an optimist is someone who looks at a pessimist and sees hope.

- **Patience.** Patience is the ability to wait and wait and wait until some sign is given that it is time to move on. Just as there is strength in motion, there is power in stillness. Western culture is big on immediate gratification, the antithesis of patience. Impatience often leads to intolerance and anger. Patience quells an angry heart.

- **Persistence.** A persistent person is someone who doesn't take no for an answer until he or she has exhausted every conceivable option. There are variations on this theme. Some people stretch the meaning of persistence to cover aggressive, in-your-face tactics. The spiritual approach is one of being pleasantly persistent (not aggressive), like flowing water that ever so slowly softens the hardest rock.

- **Resiliency.** Some people call resiliency the ability to bounce back—specifically, bouncing back from horrendous adversity. Resiliency is a trait that combines self-reliance, faith, optimism, and humor, yet resiliency is undeniably greater than the sum of these parts.

- **Unconditional love.** To extend love and compassion from your heart without conditions or expectations is the hallmark of this muscle of the soul. There are some who say that humans are not capable of unconditional love, but just ask any mother of a newborn baby and you will learn quite quickly that indeed we possess this attribute. Unconditional love is egoless.

EXERCISE **8.13**

The Hero's Journey: Exploring the Wisdom of Joseph Campbell

An ancient proverb states, "It takes a brave soul to walk the planet Earth." In the eyes of God, we are all heroes. The role of a hero is not an easy one. To depart from home can promote feelings of insecurity and even abandonment. Initiations, and there are many in one lifetime, are demanding and arduous; the phrase "baptism by fire" comes to mind. Yet through it all we are assured a warm reception upon our return, no matter the outcome of our journey.

The hero's journey is a mythical quest. Myths are clues to the spiritual potential of human life. They offer meaning and significance as well as values. A myth is a source of truth, which often becomes exaggerated, but still holds its own essence. According to Campbell, a myth does four things to assist us on this remarkable journey:

1. A myth brings us into communion with the transcendent realms and eternal forms.

2. A myth provides a revelation to waking consciousness of the power of its sustaining source.

3. A myth tells us that no matter the culture, the rituals of living and dying have spiritual and moral roots.

4. A myth fosters the centering and unfolding of the individual in integrity with the ultimate creative mystery that is both beyond and within oneself and all things.

Campbell was of the opinion that the greatest danger of the hero's journey is to fail to use the power of myth as a guide on the spiritual path. He was keenly aware that contemporary American culture has abandoned its association with myths, which is a clear and present danger to any society.

The Spiritual Quest: Your Mythical Journey

The plot of every myth includes a beginning, a middle, and an end. In this case, the beginning is a departure from the known and familiar, the middle is a set of trials (called initiations), and the end is the return home. In truth, we engage in this process of the hero's journey many times during the course of our lives.

1. **The Departure.** Are you in the process of moving out of the familiar into the unknown? What are you departing from? Some people refuse the call, often based on some fear of the unknown. Are you ignoring a call to move on?

_____

_____

_____

_____

2. **The Initiation.** The initiation is the threshold of adventure. Mythically speaking, the initiation consists of slaying a dragon or monster. In real life, initiations come in many forms, from rites of passage to issues, problems, and stressors. What is the single major life issue, concern, or problem that you are facing at the present moment?

_____

_____

_____

_____

_____

_____

3. **The Return Home.** The return is symbolized by coming home—home to the old life but with a fresh perspective. The return home bears a responsibility of sharing what you have learned on the journey. What have you learned from your most recent journey?

_____

_____

_____

_____

_____

_____

4. **A Working Myth.** What myth (source of truth) do you hold as a compass on your spiritual quest? Where did you learn this myth, and how has it helped you in your life?

_____

_____

_____

_____

_____

_____

_____

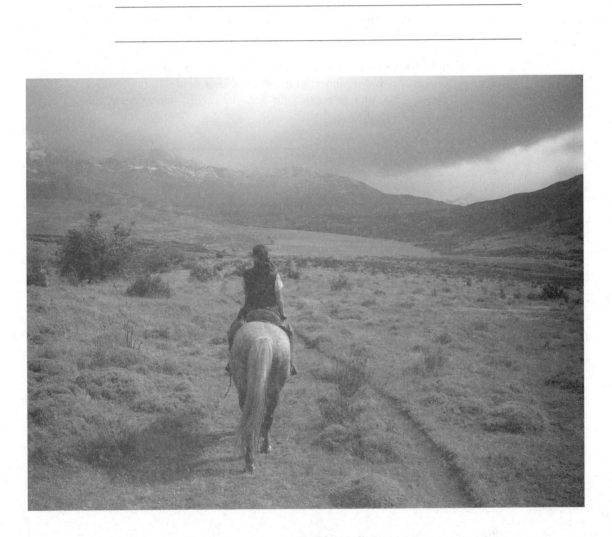

EXERCISE **8.14**

Health of the Human Spirit

Imagine, if you will, that there is a life force of divine energy that runs through your body. This life force is what we call the human spirit. We are a unique alchemy of humanity and divinity. Like a river, spirit runs through us with each breath. It is spirit that invigorates the soul. A lack of spirit can literally starve the soul, just as a lack of oxygen can starve each cell. The ways to nurture the soul are countless, yet each ensures a constant flow of this essential life force. Unresolved anger and fear are the two most common ways to choke the human spirit, yet whenever the ego dominates the soul, the health of the human spirit is diminished. The following are just a few of the many ways to enhance the health of your human spirit. As you read through these ideas, write down, in the form of lists, some ideas of what you can do to engage in these activities, and, in doing so, engage in the health of your human spirit.

1. **The Art of Self-Renewal.** Self-renewal is a practice of taking time to recharge your personal energy and reconnect to the divine source of life. List three ways in which you can find time to renew your personal energy—alone. Select the activity, the day, and the time of day.

    a. _____

    b. _____

    c. _____

2. **The Practice of Sacred Rituals.** Sacred rituals are traditions that we perform to remind us of the sacredness of life. They include any habit we engage in to which we attribute a sense of the divine. List three rituals you partake in on a regular basis to remind you of the sacredness of life.

    a. _____

    b. _____

    c. _____

3. **Embracing the Shadow.** The shadow is a symbol of our dark side, when the ego rules our lives. The shadow appears in the behaviors of prejudice, arrogance, sarcasm, and other less than desirable attributes. To embrace the shadow doesn't mean to exploit these traits, but rather to acknowledge them and work to minimize them. List three aspects of yourself that you find less than flattering. How can you begin to come to peace with these aspects of yourself?

    a. _____

    b. _____

    c. _____

4. **Acts of Forgiveness.** Forgiveness is the antidote for unresolved anger. Every act of forgiveness is an act of unconditional love. When you forgive someone, don't expect an apology. Forgiveness is not the same thing as restitution. Forgiveness is a way of letting go and moving on with your life. A large component of forgiveness is learning to forgive yourself as well. List three people who currently have made it to the top of your "s" list. First write down why you feel violated, and then write down how you can let it go and move on with your life—to forgive and start moving freely again.

a. _____

b. _____

c. _____

5. **Living Your Joy.** First, you cannot live your joy until you can name it. So, name your joy! What things in life give you pleasure—real unconditional happiness, without any sense of regret afterward? Name three things that make you happy and bring a smile to your face. Unresolved stress can inhibit the feelings of joy. List your top three pleasures. When was the last time you did each one of these? How soon can you do them again?

a. _____

b. _____

c. _____

6. **Compassion in Action.** Compassion in action is pure altruism. It is doing for others without any expectation of reciprocation. Putting compassion into action is putting the work of the soul above the priorities of the ego. Compassion in action begins as random acts of kindness, but doesn't end there. List three things you can do to express your compassion in action. Is it a random act of kindness? Is it a generous gesture? Perhaps it is just being there—without feeling a sense of obligation—really being there. Next, set out to do all three of the things on your list.

a. _____

b. _____

c. _____

EXERCISE **8.15**

Spiritual Well-Being: The Road Less Traveled

Human spirituality is so complex that it seems to defy an adequate definition or description. It is often compared to love, self-esteem, faith, and many other human characteristics that seem to be related to it. This we do know: Human spirituality involves a strong self-relationship as well as connectedness, or strong relationships with others, a strong personal value system, and a meaningful purpose in life. Unlike religions that have integrated these components, human spirituality has no rules, no dogma, and no set agenda. These concepts are related but separate entities. Psychologist Carl Jung once said, "Every crisis over the age of thirty is spiritual in nature." There is a definite relationship between stress and spirituality.

Over the years, M. Scott Peck, author of *The Road Less Traveled*, has studied the concepts of human spirituality and has developed a four-stage model to understand spiritual development. Each stage has many layers; indeed, some people seem to hover somewhere between stages. Be that as it may, these categories can help us to focus on our spiritual path.

1. **Chaotic/antisocial.** At this stage a person is manipulative, unprincipled, and governed by selfish pleasure under spiritual bankruptcy. His or her lifestyle is unorganized, in chaos or crisis, and headed for the rocks, which in turn causes much pain. All blame is externalized and projected onto others.

2. **Formal/institutional.** At this stage a sudden conversion occurs in which a person finds shelter in an institution (prison, military, or church) for security, structure, rules, and guidance. People in this stage see God as a loving but punitive figure, an "Irish cop in the sky." God is personified with human characteristics (a human face, a masculine pronoun, etc.). Institutions do, however, make some order out of the chaos.

3. **Skeptic/individual.** At this stage the person, while searching for answers, rejects the institution that claims to have them. He or she is a "born-again atheist," a person who no longer buys into the system of rules and dogma but still believes there is something out there and wants to find it. According to Peck, this is a crucial stage of development.

4. **Mystical/communal.** This is the most mature stage, when someone actively searches for new answers to life's age-old questions but feels comfortable knowing that he or she may never find the answers. A person's vision of God at this stage is as internal as it is external. Additionally, such an individual sees the need for community, or bonding, and tries to foster this. Finally, those who reach this stage realize that it is only the beginning.

Most important, spiritual well-being is an unfolding, an evolution of higher consciousness. Spirituality is also very personal; we each travel on our path at our own pace.

1. How would you define spirituality?

2. What state of well-being is your human spirit currently in?

3. In what stage of development in Peck's model do you see yourself?

4. Is your perception of God personified? Please explain.

5. Do you have a relationship with God (whatever you choose to call this and whatever you conceive it to be)? If so, how strong or weak is it? What steps could you take to improve this relationship?

_____

_____

_____

_____

_____

_____

_____

_____

_____

_____

_____

_____

_____

_____

_____

EXERCISE **8.16**

Conversations with God

How come when we talk to God, it's called praying, but when God talks to us, it's called schizophrenia?
Lily Tomlin

Recently there has been much interest in the topic of spirituality, angels, miracles, and the healing power of prayer. It could be said that we in America are going through a spiritual renaissance. One reason may be that after decades of materialistic pleasures, a large percentage of the baby-boom generation, as well as members of the so-called generation X and millennium generation, are coming up empty of any feeling of personal satisfaction. In essence, the value placed on material possessions has placed a wedge between people and their divine selves. So we find ourselves in a time of much spiritual hunger.

Although some people maintain that there is a distinction between the concepts of spirituality and religion, there is virtually no difference between the spiritual and the divine. Ideas of who or what God is may differ radically, but it is important only that you feel comfortable with your perceptions. Regardless of your conceptions, perceptions, beliefs, and attitudes, conversing with God, at some level, is the same as talking with your higher self. You might call this prayer.

Larry Dossey, M.D., has spent several years researching the concept of prayer. Like others before him who have taken a stab at understanding the divine nature of humanity, he has come to the realization that a prayer is merely a thought directed toward a power or energy that lies outside the domain of the five human senses, what Dossey calls the *non-local* mind.

Although several religions use a concept of prayer as a memorization of a poem (e.g., The Lord's Prayer, the Hail Mary) to be said in times of want or distress, this is just one of a host of ways to reach and speak to the God source that resides in and permeates all things. Prayer need not only be said in time of stress. This form of communication can be offered in times of joy and praise as well. Perhaps most important, prayer is an ongoing dialogue with your own thoughts, giving rise to the opportunity to elevate your level of consciousness by realizing your connectedness to all things. So, in actuality, all thought has prayer potential.

Prayer also reflects your relationship with that part of you which is divine. This journal theme asks you to reflect on the spiritual aspect of your health and to continue this dialogue on paper.

_____

_____

_____

_____

_____

EXERCISE **8.17**

Honoring Mother Earth

Let us think of Mother Earth.
Native American Prayer

It is no overstatement to say that the planet Earth is in trouble. It is sick and desperately fighting for survival. Water and air pollution, nuclear waste dumps, holes in the ozone, deforestation, and the incredible rate of extinction of plants and animals—the telltale signs are everywhere. All you need to do is listen to the news or read a magazine and these stories jump out and smack you across the face.

It may seem hard to believe that the earth is a living entity. Western thought, so heavily grounded in scientific ideology, makes this idea seem pagan at best. But if you were to listen to the wisdom keepers of the earth's indigenous peoples, you would hear the notion of the earth as a living entity as a sacred notion, not a foolish or ludicrous one. It is a simple truth. Even the ancient Greeks believed this, naming Mother Earth *Gaia*. Humans, once so close to the energies of the earth, have now grown very distant and separate from them. From air-conditioned bedrooms to the automobile, we have become slaves to the benefits of technology. It is not uncommon to hear people say that technology can fix what technology has damaged, which in essence puts human capabilities above the powers of the earth and sky. In the profound words of Chief Seattle, "All things connect. Man did not weave the web of life, he is merely a strand in it. Whatever he does to the web, he does to himself."

Sometimes in the cyclone of daily hassles and catastrophic events of our lives, we become disconnected from the natural elements that surround us. Whether or not we realize it, like a web, we are strongly connected to the earth. Despite all the wonderful advances in technology, we are still very dependent on the fruits and sustenance that Mother Earth provides and the cycles in which she turns. *Stress* has recently been defined as being separated or disconnected—disconnected from our friends, family, and the earth that sustains us. Inner peace is synonymous with connection and harmony with all. Therefore, part of the strategy to reduce stress is to reconnect with the planet we call home. Perhaps it's true that we can't change the world, but we can change a part of it by our interaction with it. This idea is summed up quite nicely in the slogan "Think globally, act locally."

Do some soul-searching with Mother Earth in mind. If this concept is something you have never given serious thought to, now is the time to get serious, and not in a stressful way either. Here are some questions you can ask yourself to get the ball rolling:

1. How would you best describe your relationship with the planet Earth?

2. Do you see the earth as a rock spinning in space, or as a living entity that provides sustenance in one form or another to all her species of flora and fauna?

3. Getting back to nature can take many forms, from gardening to exotic vacations. What do you do to get back to nature when the urge strikes?

4. Biological rhythms and circadian variations are constant reminders that the earth strongly influences us. Are you in touch with these rhythms and, if not, why not?

5. Any good relationship takes work. If so inclined, what steps do you feel you can take to enhance your relationship with Mother Earth?

_____

_____

_____

_____

_____

_____

_____

_____

_____

_____

_____

_____

_____

_____

_____

_____

_____

_____

_____

Effective
Coping Techniques

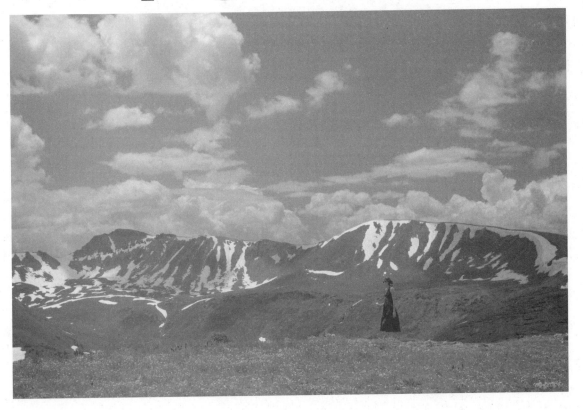

Cognitive Restructuring: Reframing

EXERCISE **9.1**

Reframing: Seeing a Bigger, Clearer Perspective

Anger and fear that arise from encountering a stressful situation can narrow our focus and distort our perspective on the bigger picture. Although the initial aspects of dealing with these situations involve some degree of grieving, the secret to coping with stress is to change the threatening perception to a nonthreatening perception. This worksheet invites you to identify three stressors and, if necessary, draft a new, "reframed" perspective (not a rationalization) that allows you to get out of the rut of a myopic view and start moving on with your life.

Example:

Situation: Can never find a parking space close to the dorm/classroom
Reframed Perspective: Although nearby parking certainly saves time, there is no denying that the walk provides much needed exercise/activity

1. Situation: _____

_____

_____

Reframed Perspective: _____

_____

_____

2. Situation: _____

_____

_____

Reframed Perspective: _____

_____

_____

3. Situation: _____

_____

_____

Reframed Perspective: _____

_____

_____

What are your mental blocks to reframing? Can you identify any?

_____

_____

Sometimes reframing works best by combining a new perspective with a symbolic image. Please revisit each example in this exercise and create a symbolic image to "lock in" the new perspective.

EXERCISE **9.2**

One Thousand Things Went Right Today!

In a stress-filled world, it becomes easy to start focusing on the negative things in life. Pretty soon you begin to attract more negative things in your life. Breaking free from this thought process isn't easy, but neither is it impossible. There is an expression, coined by Ilan Shamir, that states, "One thousand things went right today."® The concept behind this expression is that by beginning to look for the positive things in life, you will start attracting these as well—and let's face it, we could all use more positive things in our lives. Rather than taxing your mind to come up with one thousand things, or even one hundred, try starting with ten things that went right today, and then see if you can begin to include this frame of mind at the midpoint of each day to keep you on course. Remember, in a world of negativity, it takes work to be happy!

1. _____

2. _____

3. _____

4. _____

5. _____

6. _____

7. _____

8. _____

9. _____

10. _____

After having written down these things, is there any lesson that comes to mind that you can learn from this experience?

_____

_____

_____

_____

_____

_____

_____

_____

_____

_____

_____

_____

_____

_____

_____

_____

_____

_____

_____

_____

_____

_____

_____

_____

_____

_____

EXERCISE **9.3**

Positive Affirmation Statements

Positive affirmation statements are thoughts or expressions that you can repeat to your-self to boost your self-esteem. These words of inspiration highlight the positive as-pects of your own personality that enhance and nurture your self-esteem. They are expressions that build confidence, provide inspiration, lift the spirit to rise above mediocrity, and help you function at your highest human potential.

It is easy to give yourself negative feedback about almost anything. We each have a critic who metaphorically sits on our shoulder and whispers negative thoughts in our ear. The media do this too, striking at our insecurities through subliminal and overt advertising with over fifteen hundred messages per day. In addition, we often in-terpret feedback to be negative from family, friends, and other people who pass in and out of our lives. But worst of all, perhaps as a learned behavior, we continually feed ourselves negative thoughts, which continually deflate self-esteem.

Using positive affirmation statements is really a behavior modification tech-nique that, in conjunction with relaxation techniques (deep breathing or mental im-agery), trains the mind to give the battered ego positive strokes and strengthen self-esteem. Although there are no specific rules, there are some guidelines that can make these positive affirmations work for you: (1) Phrase your affirmation in the pres-ent tense, such as "I am a lovable person." (2) Phrase your affirmation in the most positive way. (3) Make your affirmation simple, clear, and precise. (4) Choose an affir-mation that feels right for you.

The following list is a sample of some positive affirmation statements that others have used for this purpose. A positive affirmation statement should be a personal thought or expression. However, if you cannot think of one right away, feel free to use one or more of these. Eventually, you may want to take a moment to think of one that is personal. Positive affirmation statements should be somewhat short—something you can repeat to yourself in one breath.

Damn, I'm good!

I am one with the Tao.

Love is the answer.

I am calm and relaxed.

I have confidence in myself.

I am an important piece of the whole.

I am a lovable person.

I radiate success.

I am worthy of being loved.

I am the source of my happiness and security.

Your Affirmation Statement:

_____

Because the unconscious mind needs to be involved with this process, and the unconscious mind doesn't use words to communicate, it is best to combine your affirmation statement with an image or symbol to unite both minds for the best effect. Select a symbolic image (e.g., a rose, a small reflective pond, an eagle, or a rainbow) and describe it here:

_____

Now that you have chosen your positive affirmation statement, write down ten places or times of day that you can say it to yourself to reinforce this message. Then do it!

Places to Use Your Affirmation Statement and Symbol

1. _____

2. _____

3. _____

4. _____

5. _____

6. _____

7. _____

8. _____

9. _____

10. _____

EXERCISE **9.4**

Optimist or Pessimist?

You should always be aware that your head creates your world.
Ken Keyes

Within each person resides the makings of an optimist and pessimist. Some people claim dominion of their optimist side, always seeing the glass as half full, whereas others clearly see themselves as pessimists, viewing the glass as half empty (or, in some cases, completely empty). Most people see themselves as being somewhere in between depending on a variety of life circumstances, although in general we tend to gravitate toward one side or the other in our worldview. Describe the difference between an optimist and a pessimist in your opinion, and give an example of each. Then explain on which side you see yourself most of the time and why.

_____

_____

_____

_____

_____

_____

_____

_____

_____

_____

_____

_____

_____

_____

EXERCISE **9.5**

The Things I Take for Granted

Almost instinctively, human beings have given thanks since they first set foot on earth. From animal sacrifices to banquet feasts to silent moments of praise, showing appreciation for everything from the smallest of gifts to some of life's greatest pleasures is very much a part of the human condition. Before televised football games and New York City parades, a unique tradition was established on the shores of the New World several hundred years ago when English immigrants and Native Americans sat down to perhaps the most famous autumn feast ever created, Thanksgiving; appropriately, it became a yearly event in America.

It is easy to give thanks and praise in time of joy and happiness. Giving thanks is rarely thought of, however, in times of crisis. Actually, stress can produce some very ungrateful attitudes. Stressful events tend to cloud the mind with thoughts of frustration and anguish—some directed inward, most directed outward—and these can leave little room for anything else. When the Pilgrims sat down to the first turkey dinner, times were hard. There was no indoor plumbing; there were no drug stores, no credit cards, and no daycare centers. Life was a real challenge. But in that challenge life was reduced to the simplest of terms: survival. In our day and age, survival is pretty much a given. The question isn't "Will I survive?" but rather "How well can I live?" Although theoretically the high-tech age has improved the quality of life, it also seems to bring with it pressures that negate this standard of quality.

More stress and less time to enjoy life's simple pleasures can often make it difficult to take adequate time to sit back every now and then and appreciate the little things that make life special. Stress can act as blinders to our field of vision. By consciously taking these blinders off, we can see the whole picture in better focus. Taking things for granted is as much a part of human nature as giving thanks. Often, we don't know what we have until it's gone. A list of things that you take for granted could be endless. But if you were to stop and think for a moment about what some of these might include, just what would they be and why?

EXERCISE **9.6**

Healthy Pleasures

In their book *Healthy Pleasures*, Robert Ornstein and David Sobel discuss the idea that in order to create a sense of balance in our lives, we need to remind ourselves to pat ourselves on the back, take responsibility for our moments of happiness, and engage in a host of behaviors that bring us a sense of joy and satisfaction. Listing healthy pleasures also helps steer you in the direction of positive psychology.

Now you may say, "Hey, I already do this!" But most people don't, especially after they get out of college and get caught up in making money, paying bills, raising kids, and taking care of parents.

Healthy pleasures are just that: healthy. They don't cost much, either. To look at a sunset, to take an early morning walk in the woods, to treat yourself to an ice cream cone—these are healthy pleasures. How quickly they are forgotten when we feel stressed!

This exercise asks you to list 25 healthy pleasures that you participate in on a regular basis. If you cannot come up with 25, list things you consider healthy pleasures that you intend to do soon.

1. _____

2. _____

3. _____

4. _____

5. _____

6. _____

7. _____

8. _____

9. _____

10. _____

11. _____

12. _____

13. _____

14. _____

15. _____

16. _____

17. _____

18. _____

19. _____

20. _____

21. _____

22. _____

23. _____

24. _____

25. _____

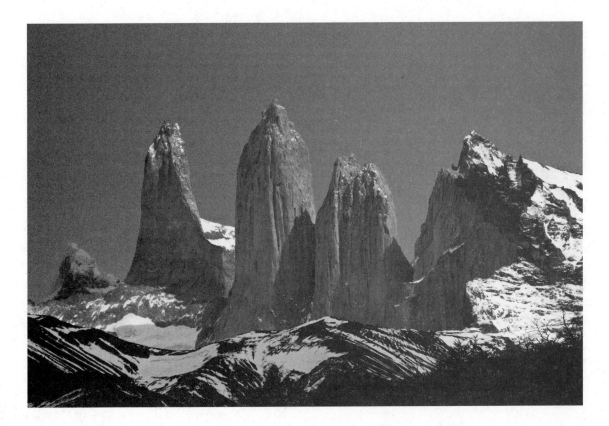

Behavior Modification

EXERCISE **10.1**

Value Assessment and Clarification

Values—those abstract ideals that shape our lives—are important constructs. They give the conscious mind structure. They can also give countries and governments structure. The U.S. Declaration of Independence is all about values, including "life, liberty, and the pursuit of happiness." Although values are intangible, they are often symbolized by material objects or possessions, which can make values very real. Some everyday examples of values are love, peace, privacy, education, freedom, happiness, creativity, fame, integrity, faith, friendship, morals, health, justice, loyalty, honesty, and independence.

Where do values come from? We adopt values at a very early age, unconsciously, from people we admire, love, or desire acceptance from, such as our parents, brothers and sisters, school teachers, and clergy. Values are often categorized into two groups: *basic* values, a collection of three to five instrumental values that are the cornerstones of the foundation of our personalities, and *supporting* values, which augment our basic values. Throughout our development we construct a value system, a collection of values that influences our attitudes and behaviors, all of which make up our personality. If you are not sure what your values are, look to see where you spend your time and money.

As we mature, our value systems also change because we become accountable for the way we think and behave. Like the earth's tectonic plates, our values shift in importance, causing our own earth to quake. These shifts are called *value conflicts*, and they can cause a lot of stress. Classic examples of value conflicts include love versus religious faith or social class (Romeo and Juliet), freedom versus responsibility, and work versus leisure (the American Dream). Conflicts in values can be helpful in our own maturing process if we work through the conflict to a full resolution. Problems arise when we ignore the conflict and avoid clarifying our value system. The purpose of this journal theme is for you to take an honest look at your value system, assess its current status, and clarify unresolved issues associated with values in conflict. The following are some questions to help you in the process of values assessment and clarification.

1. Make a list of the core values you hold. (Values come from things that give you meaning and importance, yet they are abstract in nature.)

2. See if you can identify which of these values are basic, or instrumental, at this point in your life and which support or augment your basic values.

3. How are your values represented in your possessions? (For example, a BMW may represent wealth or freedom.)

4. Describe how your values influence your dominant thoughts, attitudes, and beliefs.

5. Do you have any values that compete for priority with one another? If so, what are they, and why is there a conflict?

6. What do you see as the best way to begin to resolve this conflict in values? Ask yourself whether it is time to change the priority of your values or perhaps discard values that no longer give importance to your life.

Peace & Relaxation

① 1.1 (pg 3)   suprised that 12 - high
   2.1 (pg k)   considered
                   feels like "maintenance"

                   13 yes / 21 No   1 16
                                                              33
        2.7   1   9
   Chpt 5 5.1   ✓   _____
②   6   6.6   ✓   5 8

   7.2 83.84   8.2   ⑤ ?No
   7.3
③   Mod 8 29
   8.14 (124)   Chpt 28
                                                      exer. 28.5
   10.2 Behaviors i'd like to △   pg 278
   ⊕ try something
            arthstic -   } results/thoughts
   what did I
        do - how do
           I feel? helpful
④   or not

⑥   Mod 7.
   Red   excl to use-   chp 22 music
   Scared   dont anywhere;   therapy
   18 19 20 21   no equip. pain   cerful to
                                               ① 76
   diaphragmatic   ② p13
       breathing
                                            23.2 try T time
   19.1 exercise   helpful?
                                            (compare to trad massage?)
   Chpt 21 - try
        guided
           imagry
              is
          useful
          for me?
          for pts?

EXERCISE **10.2**

Behaviors I'd Like to Change

If one desires change, one must be that change first before that change can take place.
Gita Bellin

If you are like most people, you seek some type of self-improvement on a regular basis. Perhaps it's something you notice yourself doing. The catalyst for change may more likely be a suggestion from a friend or, worse, someone of whom you aren't too particularly fond. The most recognized time to make behavioral changes is January 1, when the year is new, the slate is clean, and the winds of change are in the air. Another time that we are reminded to make changes is on or around our birthdays— again, a clean slate.

Two types of personalities and the respective behaviors linked with stress have now become household words: Type A and codependency. Type A behaviors include compulsive actions related to urgency, supercompetitiveness, and hostile aggression. These characteristics, primarily feelings of unresolved hostility, are thought to be closely associated with coronary heart disease. Codependent behaviors include perfectionism, overachievement, ardent approval seeking, control of others, inability to express anger and other feelings, ardent loyalty to loved ones, and overreactions. These types of behaviors are now strongly linked to cancer. The newest personality type associated with stress is called Type D, which relates to depression caused by unresolved anger issues.

Sometimes we are aware of our behaviors, but many times we are not. These actions are so ingrained in us that they are often second nature, so we seldom give them thought. Only when something we do is pointed out to us, or in an unguarded moment, do we see ourselves as perhaps others see us.

Behavioral psychologists have come to agree that changes are made first through awareness and then through motivation to change. But changing several habits at one time, which usually people try to do at the start of each new year, is very difficult, if not impossible. What is now commonly suggested is to try to change one behavior at a time. This way there is a greater chance of accomplishment. The following progression of steps, when followed, can augment this process of behavioral change.

1. Become aware of your current behavior (e.g., biting one's fingernails).

2. Find a new mindset to precede the new behavior you want to introduce (e.g., biting my nails is bad and I need to stop doing this).

3. Substitute a more desirable behavior in place of the old one (e.g., in the act of biting nails, stop and take a few deep breaths to relax).

4. Evaluate the outcome of trying the new behavior and renew or revise your plan and commitment (e.g., deep breathing helped, especially on that date last night; I'll keep trying this).

Sometimes it helps to write these steps down. Do you have any behaviors that you wish to modify or change? What are your options? Sketch them out here!

_____

_____

_____

_____

_____

_____

_____

_____

_____

_____

_____

_____

_____

_____

_____

_____

_____

_____

_____

_____

EXERCISE **10.3**

Assertiveness Training 101

Please write your initial reaction to each of the situations described below, followed by a more assertive response if necessary.

Part I
Situation 1: A Failed Exam

You receive a failing grade on the first exam in a course for your major, and you are devastated. You feel as if the grade is not a true reflection of your knowledge of the subject.

Initial Reaction: _____

_____

_____

Assertive Response: _____

_____

_____

Situation 2: Poor Boundaries

You come home from class or work starved, only to discover that one of your room-mates has eaten your food (again). You are on a limited budget and cannot feed the world.

Initial Reaction: _____

_____

_____

Assertive Response: _____

_____

_____

Situation 3: Strong-Back Favors

One of your best college friends has to move out of his apartment at the end of the month and has found a new place to live a few miles away. He tells you that he really needs some help moving and needs to borrow a car like yours. He asks for both your time and your car. You have two term papers due immediately after the same weekend.

Initial Reaction: _____

_____

_____

Assertive Response: _____

_____

_____

Any additional thoughts:

_____

_____

_____

_____

_____

_____

_____

Part II

1. Select an undesirable behavior that you are aware you perform (e.g., drinking expensive designer coffee).

    _____

    _____

    _____

    _____

2. Ask yourself how motivated you are to change this behavior. (Remember: As with any change, there might be sacrifices involved.) Ask yourself whether the costs of making this change will outweigh the benefits.

    _____

    _____

    _____

3. Think about what changes in your perceptions and attitudes must accompany this behavioral change, and how you can adopt these new perceptions as your own to become second nature.

_____

_____

_____

4. Specify what new behavior you wish to adopt. It is best not to think of stating that you want to stop the old behavior (a negative thought process). The new behavior should be expressed as a positive goal (e.g., "I would like to have long fingernails").

_____

_____

_____

5. After trying the new behavior, ask yourself how you did. Was your first or second attempt successful? Why or why not? If not, what other approaches can you take to accomplish this goal?

_____

_____

_____

EXERCISE **10.4**

Healthy Boundaries

We are living in an age in which the average person has very poor boundaries in his or her life. Technology may be a factor, but it's not the only reason. People bring their work home, while at the same time problems from home invade their professional lives. It seems as if almost everyone has poor financial boundaries, with the average person carrying well over $3,000 annually in credit card debt. People think nothing of bringing their cell phones into college classrooms, restaurants, and movie theaters, and what begins as just an hour in front of the television ends up being a whole evening. Poor personal boundaries result in feelings of being overwhelmed, annoyed, and victimized—all of which contribute to a critical mass of stress.

First, healthy boundaries require an insight about what's appropriate in each and every setting in which you find yourself—in essence, creating the boundaries you need and want to maintain a sense of personal balance. Next, healthy boundaries require courage to assert your boundaries so that they are not violated. Finally, healthy boundaries require willpower and discipline to honor what you yourself have established, in order to give you better structure and stability in your life.

1. List four areas in your life that you feel have weak boundaries (or perhaps no boundaries). Examples might include finances, alcohol, technology, or television watching.

    a. _____

    b. _____

    c. _____

    d. _____

2. Now, please list four boundaries that you would like to create in your life to bring about a sense of balance. Then add a few words about what you can do to have these boundaries honored.

    a. _____

    b. _____

    c. _____

    d. _____

EXERCISE **10.5**

Reinventing Yourself (Again)

We enter this world with a clean slate, yet from the first day, our behaviors and mishaps and, later, our accomplishments (or lack thereof) begin to define who we are to everyone we meet and know. Through our thoughts, words, and actions we paint a composite image that we present to the world. As we mature from teenagers to adults, many of the things we did in our early years serve as a constant reminder of mistakes or poor judgments made along the way. And there are always people (such as our parents) who remember us as we were, not as we have become.

Going to college provides a great means to wipe the slate clean again and start anew. New people, new friends, and new relationships lay the foundation for a refined image of who we are evolving into. Reinventing yourself is best described as taking your best qualities and building on them. Reinventing yourself is not running away from all your troubles and worries and pretending to be someone you are not. Instead, reinventing yourself is maturing your finest qualities and leaving behind those aspects that don't serve your highest good. Of course, it really helps when you can do this in a new environment where the slate is truly clean. Al Gore reinvented himself. Lance Armstrong reinvented himself. So did Martha Stewart. You can too.

Here is the catch to reinventing yourself: You have to start from the ground up. This means that you have to know in your mind how you want to be, how you want to act. Reinventing yourself begins in the mind long before it manifests itself in your actions. In simple terms, reinventing yourself means adapting to a new situation.

Who reinvents themselves? Retirees, college graduates, empty-nest moms, released convicts. Practically everyone. Are you in a position to reinvent yourself?

Why would you want to reinvent yourself? Simple! Perhaps you have been attracting the wrong kind of person in your intimate relationships. Perhaps you keep finding yourself in the same kind of meaningless job. There are many reasons.

So if you were in the frame of mind to reinvent yourself, where would you start? Attitude, food, clothes, movies, music, haircut, or all of the above? Knowing that reinventing yourself begins in the mind, consider that your slate is now clean. Describe how you would like to see the new and improved you.

_____

_____

_____

_____

_____

_____

_____

Make a list of ten things you can do to create the new and improved you.

1. _____

2. _____

3. _____

4. _____

5. _____

6. _____

7. _____

8. _____

9. _____

10. _____

Chapter 11

Journal Writing

EXERCISE 11.1

Unwritten Letters

Many times we wish to communicate with someone we love, like, or just know well, but for one reason or another—whether it be anger, procrastination, or not finding the right words at the right time—we part ways without fully resolving those special feelings. There was once a college student whose former boyfriend took his life. In the note left behind, he specifically mentioned her, and the words haunted her for what seemed like an eternity. As a result of counseling, she decided to write him a letter to express her feelings of anger, sorrow, loneliness, and love. Through her words, her letter began the resolution process and ultimately her path toward inner peace.

This theme of resolution through letter writing has been the subject of many books, plays, and movies. In a movie made for television entitled *Message to My Daughter*, a young mother with a newborn baby discovers she has terminal cancer. As a part of her resolution process, she records several cassette tapes with personal messages to her daughter. Many father-son relationships also fall into this category when emotional distance becomes a nearly impassable abyss. Years later, a movie titled *My Life*, starring Michael Keaton, had a similar plot. It is a common theme.

It has been said that with recent advances in technology, from the cell phone to the microchip, Americans are writing fewer and fewer personal letters. Sociologists worry that future generations will look back on this time period, the information high-tech age, and never really know what individuals were actually feeling and thinking because there will be few, if any, written entries to trace these perceptions. Moreover, psychologists agree that many of today's patients are troubled and unable to articulate their thoughts and feelings completely, which leaves them with feelings of unresolved stress.

This journal entry concerns the theme of resolution. The following are some suggestions that might inspire you to draft a letter to someone you have been meaning to write. Now is your chance.

1. Compose a letter to someone to whom you were close who has passed away or someone you haven't been in contact with for a long time. Tell that person what you have been up to, perhaps any major changes in your life, or changes that you foresee occurring in the months or years ahead. If you have any unresolved feelings toward this person, try expressing them in appropriately crafted words so that you can resolve these feelings and come to a sense of lasting peace.

2. Write a letter to yourself. Imagine that you have one month to live. What would you do in these last thirty days? Assume that there are no limitations. Who would you see? Where would you visit? What would you do? Why?

3. Pretend that you now have a baby. What would you like to share with your son or daughter now, should, for some reason, you not have the opportunity to do so later in life? What would you like your child to know about you? For example, perhaps you would share things that you wanted to know about your parents or grandparents, which now are pieces missing in your life.

4. Write a letter to anyone you wish for whatever reason. If you need additional space to write, use the extra pages provided at the back of the book.

EXERCISE **11.2**

The Vision Quest

Our lives are a series of events strung together through the spirit of each breath and heartbeat. Some events are more significant than others because they mark powerful changes in the growth and development of our existence. In earlier cultures, as far back as the dawn of humankind, these events of change, these transitions from one life stage to another, were referred to as *rites of passage*. These rites often included a ceremony of celebration. Today, these rites are often continued in such practices as bar mitzvahs, weddings, baby showers, and funerals.

In modern American culture, the importance of personal rites of passage has been de-emphasized or forgotten. Attention is placed on the ceremony without true recognition of its purpose. In reality, many of our major life events are done alone with no supportive guidance, no community involvement, and no celebration. Modern technology has also replaced our sense of origin, leaving us uncentered and ungrounded. The result often leaves us unable to deal effectively with the stress produced from life's crises or without the maturity to advance through the developmental stages of life.

In the tradition of the Native American, a vision quest marks a significant rite of passage. It is a wilderness retreat where one reflects on one's inner resources as well as reaffirms one's centeredness and connection to Mother Earth. In a vision quest, the individual seeks a vision of a meaningful purpose in life and gains a greater understanding of himself or herself from within. This concept has been adopted as a cornerstone of the nation's Outward Bound program: self-reliance through introspection in nature.

A vision quest marks a major life transition. Those who initiate this quest search for a vision to guide them through the transitional period of change. Although in the truest sense a vision quest is done in the solitude of the wilderness, you can initiate this process anywhere. As you work through these questions, note the similarity between these stages and the stages of Joseph Campbell's hero's journey. The following questions are provided to lead you on the first steps of your vision quest.

1. What significant events to date would you consider to be rites of passage in your life? Why do you consider these to be rites of passage for you?

2. Take a moment to ask yourself what life event you are in the midst of. What dragons are you battling with right now? What life passage are you entering or emerging from? Rites of passage are thought to have three distinct phases. As you ponder these questions, follow these phases of the vision quest:

   a. **Severance:** A separation from old ways—from a familiar lifestyle, habits, and perhaps even people.

   b. **Threshold:** The actual quest, a search for a vision or understanding of this transition, an inventory of inner resources and external surroundings to provide guidance through the transition period.

c. **Incorporation:** A return from the quest to the community, with new insight and the ability to apply the knowledge from this experience as you progress in the development of your life.

3. During a vision quest, one receives the gift of a name to symbolize connectedness and groundedness. What name does the wind whisper in your ears?

_____

_____

_____

_____

_____

_____

_____

_____

_____

_____

_____

_____

_____

_____

_____

_____

_____

_____

Source: Brian Luke Seaward, _Managing Stress: A Creative Journal_ (Boston: Jones and Bartlett Publishers, 2004).

EXERCISE **11.3**

The Key to Consciousness (The Key to Your Heart)

Note: Before you start this journal writing exercise, please consider going to a hardware store and purchasing an uncut house designer key (about $2).

The story of Pandora's box is a metaphor of the human mind: a symbolic rendering of the fact that, when unlocked, the mind offers a direct but often cluttered path to one's heart. Legend tells us that the treasure box sat undisturbed for ages because humanity was warned never to open it for fear that dangerous things might escape. When it was finally opened (out of curiosity's sake), many things did indeed escape—metaphors for unresolved issues of anger and fear (thoughts and emotions kept secret from the conscious mind for ages, yet thoughts and deep-seated emotions that greatly influence our behavior). The one thing that was kept locked in Pandora's box, the one aspect that was denied freedom in order to help resolve the issues of anger and fear, was hope: hope for a better world. It is that hope we are here to access today. Hope for a better life, for a balanced life, for a clean healthy heart, and for a better world in which to navigate our lives.

We hold many secrets in the depths of our unconscious mind—secrets from our childhood, teen years, and even our early adult years that greatly influence, for better (or more likely worse), our current lifestyle. Some might say that secrets hold us prisoner from a better, more liberating life. How does one unlock the doors of the unconscious mind? How does one set oneself free from the chains of the past? First, it takes the desire to uncover these secrets and deal with whatever issues need resolution. Next, it takes the courage to pick up the key, place it in the lock, turn it, and open it. This lock is the complex security system of the ego. As a means of protection, the ego makes great efforts to keep these secrets secret, meaning that it is very hard to release them and work to resolve them. Difficult, yes, but not impossible. Every treasure holds a peril. But every issue also holds a valuable lesson—when we take the time to resolve it and learn from it.

Every groove, every cut, every knob on a cut key, is there for a reason. No two locks are alike; hence, every key is unique! The key in your hand is uncut. No one can cut the grooves but you. Holding this key in your hand, take some time to examine the symbolic lock into which it fits. With the power of your imagination, as you explore the landscape of your unconscious mind, make the necessary cuts and grooves in this unique key so that it becomes functional as a means to open the deeper layers of your mind. This is your key to hope, your key to spiritual freedom.

What will happen when you take off the lock and open the door to your unconscious mind? What will you find there? This soul-searching exercise is an invitation to delve into your unconscious mind and make peace with these secrets, unveil them, and then release them so that you may find a new sense of freedom in your life—a life supported in hope and realized in love and compassion.

EXERCISE **11.4**

A Gift from the Sea

Individuals are each very different, yet we all share many common features, thoughts, even perceptions. Our makeup is complex, yet similar from one person to another. We all have qualities that we consider either strengths or weaknesses, and these certainly vary from person to person. Strengths can be magnified to bolster self-esteem. Weaknesses, too, can be magnified and become roadblocks to our human potential. The world is full of metaphors regarding the facets of our lives. For example, a seashell can be considered a metaphor, a symbol of ourselves.

After an extremely stressful event that changed the life of Anne Morrow Lindbergh and her husband, Charles, Anne took refuge on a secluded beach to find peace of mind and solace in her heart. In her book *Gift from the Sea*, Lindbergh shares her personal thoughts as she cradled a series of seashells in the palms of her hands and reflected on the images they suggested, as well as on the symbolism each offered.

The following thoughts and questions inspired by Lindbergh's book are provided to help you explore this shell metaphor. You don't need to have a seashell in hand to do this exercise, but sometimes something tangible can really open up your thoughts.

1. Pick a shell from a collection of shells (real or imaginary) and hold it in your hand for a moment. Close your eyes and really feel it. What was it that attracted you to this particular shell? Take a moment to describe the shell you picked: its color, shape, texture, and size.

2. Many sea creatures have shells. Some have beautifully colored shells and some have incredible detail with ridges, points, and curls. Some shells are quite small, whereas others are very big. Some shells are very fragile, whereas others seem the epitome of strength. Like sea creatures, we too have shells, though they are not quite as obvious. What is your shell like? Describe its shape, color, texture, and any other features that you wish to include—features that differentiate it from other shells.

3. A shell serves a purpose for a sea creature. It acts as a home as well as a form of protection—a base for security. The shells we have also act as a means of protection. Our shells, too, can offer a form of strength and security, but they can also overprotect. Does your own shell overprotect, or is it a growing shell?

4. We all have strengths and weaknesses. Strengths are strong points of our personality or attributes that bring us favorable attention. Weaknesses, on the other hand, are what we perceive as our faults, insecurities, or attributes that we associate with negative connotations. List your strengths and beside this list write your weaknesses. Now take a careful look at this list. Sometimes strengths can actually be weaknesses, while some weaknesses can be disguised

as our strong points. For example, take a person who is well organized. This could be considered a weakness if it spills over into perfectionism. Sometimes what we see as our weaknesses others see as our strengths, and this may in fact be true. Many times it is the perceptions that make this difference. Now take a look at your list again. Are any of your strengths potential weaknesses or vice versa?

5. Feel free to add any comments, feelings, and even memories to this journal entry.

_____

_____

_____

_____

_____

_____

_____

_____

_____

_____

_____

_____

_____

_____

_____

_____

_____

Source: Brian Luke Seaward, *Managing Stress: A Creative Journal* (Boston: Jones and Bartlett Publishers, 2004).

EXERCISE **11.5**

The Seed

Begin this journal exercise with a seed (walnut, sunflower, tulip bulb, poppy, etc.). Hold the seed in your hand and close your eyes for a moment. Within your hand is a seed, the gift of life. Within this seed is a powerhouse of creation. From the tiniest seed grows the largest tree. From large seeds grow flowers, fruits, and an abundance of gifts that exult the five senses. The seed is the quintessential metaphor that represents the multitude of ideas or possibilities within each and every one of us. Inside each seed is the coded wisdom to manifest our intentions, whatever they may happen to be—but only if the right conditions exist.

If seeds are like ideas, intentions, or prayers that we cast out to the four winds in the hopes of taking root, then our minds are similar to the fields of earth that await the collaboration of creativity. A seed that lands on unfertile soil is no different than an idea that finds its way into one's own inhospitable mind. Doubts, fears, frustrations, attachments, and conditional desires often sabotage the potential of each seed ready to germinate.

1. Using the seed as a metaphor, comb the recesses of your heart to come up with one intention that you truly wish to manifest in your life. Like the seed that you hold in your hand, describe it in fine detail.

2. Like the tree from which the seed came, take a moment to reflect on the source of your inspiration. Where did your intention originate? By gaining clarity on this, you create a stronger bond of energy from source to seed, thereby ensuring a stronger outcome.

3. Just as there are many natural (and unnatural) things that can impede the growth of the seed that hits the ground, so too there are impeding thoughts within our own mind that can sterilize the strongest seeds. By recognizing these factors, we can begin to take steps to cleanse the ground and refertilize it for the best effect. What thoughts inhibit the growth of your best intentions?

4. In the best words possible, visualize the realization of your intention, not only the roots, but the branches and leaves as well. In essence, what fruit will this seed bear when it is fully grown?

_____

EXERCISE **11.6**

From a Distance

Sometimes when we distance ourselves from our problems, we get a different and perhaps more objective viewpoint of our perceptions. Looking at ourselves through someone else's eyes gives us a chance to detach from our emotions long enough to find a new way to deal with the problem. When people write journal entries, they write almost exclusively in the first person (*I*). This first-person viewpoint is often what separates autobiographical truth from a third-person point of view, which is often incomplete because it lacks significant personal insight. But let us assume for a moment that an occasional journal entry could be written in the third person (*she, he*). Imagine what could be revealed using that unique insight that only you could provide, but with the objectivity of a third person with no emotional attachment—the best of both worlds.

A journal entry of this nature would read like a story or screenplay. It would have a plot (your stressor of the day); it would have character development (your thoughts and feelings that this observer described); it would have mystery (how to resolve the stressor); and it might even have adventure and romance—but let's not get carried away. Save this journal entry for when you have had a really bad day or your mind has been weighed down so heavily that you just cannot be objective with your thoughts; then pull out a pen and write about this concern from the perspective of someone else looking at the situation. You'll be surprised at just how therapeutic and revealing this type of entry can be.

_____

_____

_____

_____

_____

_____

_____

_____

_____

_____

EXERCISE **11.7**

Lessons Learned

Is it possible that life is one big schoolroom or that the planet Earth is a laboratory for learning? There are many people who believe so. But unlike the structural classrooms that we attend from kindergarten through graduate school, the classroom of life is virtually experimental in nature. Moreover, there are neither grades nor curves. There are no diplomas, just a wealth of accumulated knowledge that we call *wisdom*.

The school of life does not require studying in the form of memorization as much as it necessitates a continual synthesis of information and our experiences. The goal of our individual lesson plan is to discover the universal truths and to apply these in the framework of our lives. Each experience has a lesson to offer if we choose to take the time to learn from it. As with other forms of schooling, there are times when we play hooky and miss out on important material. In the end, our lives are an open book in which we write the lessons we've learned.

Some of life's lessons are so obvious that we walk right through, missing them completely. Others are so painful that we choose to avoid them. However, through it all we are very much aware, either consciously or unconsciously, of the meaning of our experiences. An ancient Chinese proverb states, "When the pupil is ready, the teacher will come," meaning that when we take the time to explore the purpose of our life experiences, we will understand, and the lessons will be learned. To be "ready" is to be still with thought, allowing the mind liberty to interpret the meaning of these lessons.

Before you start this journal theme, you might want to sit comfortably, close your eyes for a moment, and relax. Take a few deep breaths and begin to clear your mind of any distracting thoughts. Then use the following questions to ready the student within yourself so that the teacher may come.

1. What would you say is the most valuable of all the lessons that you have learned in your life to date?

2. What events led to this experience?

3. What was it that sparked this moment of revelation?

4. Are there any experiences that you still question the meaning of?

5. What events that have caused you pain and that you are avoiding may ultimately bear the fruit of understanding once resolved?

6. Finally, there is an expression that says, "To know and not to do is not to know." Are there some lessons you thought you had learned and then forgot to apply in your life that caused history to repeat itself? If so, what were they? Do you have any other comments you wish to add?

Chapter 12

Expressive Art Therapy

EXERCISE 12.1

The Human Butterfly

Theme: The butterfly is a symbol of transformation, of rising above life's issues and problems and moving on. The words for "butterfly" and "soul" are synonymous in Greek.

Activity: Spread out some colored crayons or pastels on a table or floor area where you can easily access them. If you are doing this with others, please remember to share! Allocate about ten to fifteen minutes to color in the wings of your butterfly (see the accompanying figure). As an additional phase of the human butterfly exercise, consider writing in the butterfly wings those inner resources or muscles of the soul (e.g., humor, patience, forgiveness, creativity, optimism) that you use to effectively cope with problems. If there are inner resources that you feel you would like to have be a stronger part of who you are (to enhance your coping skills), then write those attributes on the outside of the butterfly and draw arrows from the words into the wing of the butterfly. By doing so, you send a direct message to your unconscious mind to begin to utilize these inner resources more often.

Interpretation: If you do this exercise in a small group, take turns showing your butterfly illustration and explain to the group your best interpretation from an archetypal perspective. When viewing other's work, you cannot help but be impressed, if for no other reason then seeing how different and unique each butterfly is when colored.

Outside Assignments: Consider hanging your butterfly on the fridge or office wall as a means to remind you (both consciously and unconsciously) of your inner resources.

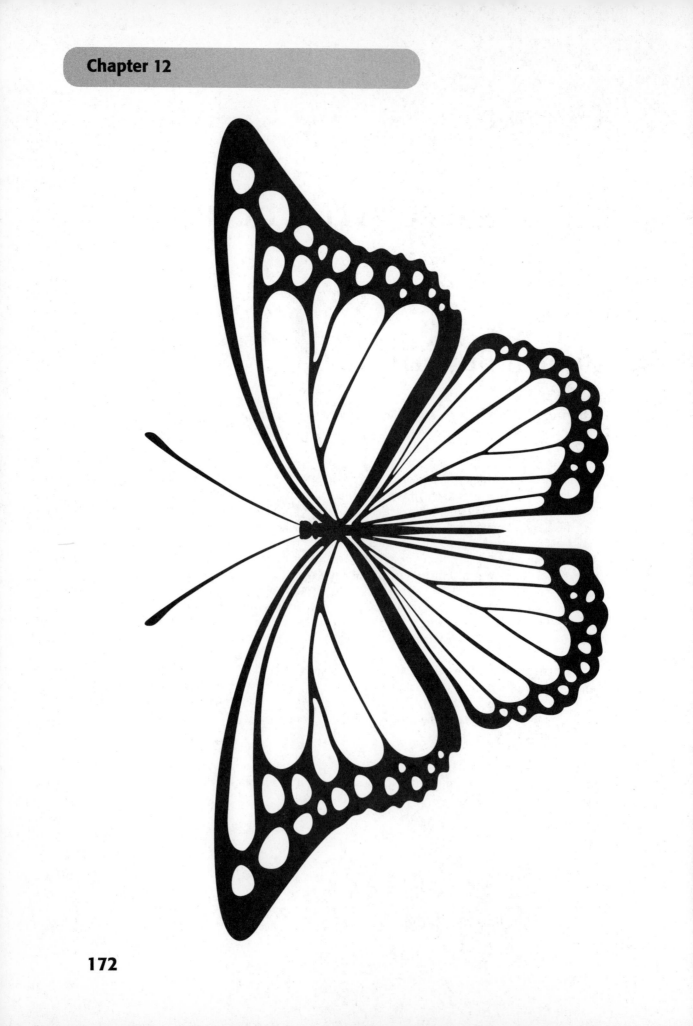

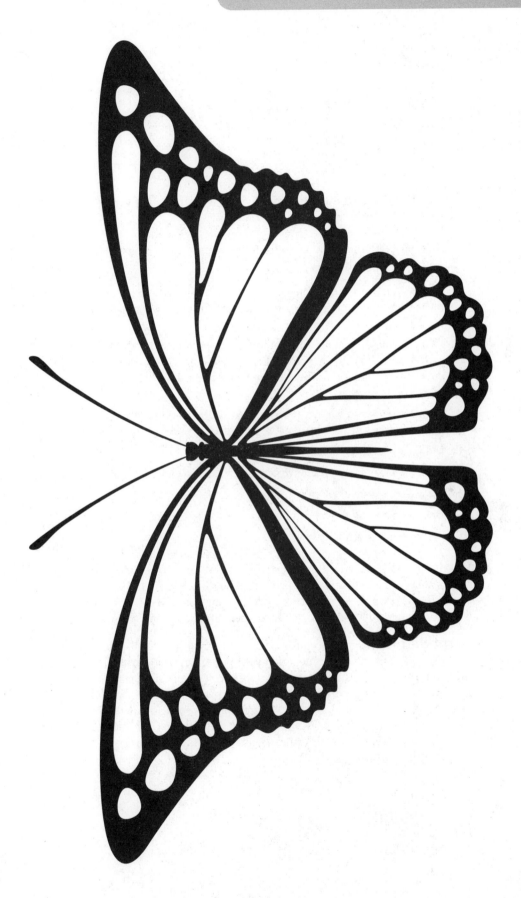

EXERCISE **12.2**

Beyond Words: Drawing for Emotional Relief

Art Therapy Themes: The following is a list of popular themes in the field of art therapy from which to choose.

1. Draw an expression of how you feel when you are either angry or afraid.

2. Draw a sketch of yourself (how you see yourself).

3. Closing your eyes, draw a line on the paper. Then open your eyes and slowly rotate the paper around until an image appears from which to continue and finish the sketch.

4. In the theme of healing, draw an actual or representational illustration of a part of your body that is not whole (e.g., because of disease or illness). Then, draw a second image in which healing has occurred. (It's very important to do this second image.)

5. Draw a mandala (a circular personal coat of arms with four quadrants depicting four aspects of your life that are important to you).

6. Draw your favorite animal.

7. Draw an image from a recent (or vivid) dream or recurring dream.

8. Draw a significant event in your life.

9. Draw a house (either one you live in or perhaps wish to live in).

10. Draw whatever you wish!

Instructions: Please read through the list of themes and then select one and begin to create your piece of artwork, spending about fifteen to twenty minutes for this exercise. If time permits, you might consider selecting a second theme, which then allows you to choose which drawing to share when done as a group activity.

Interpretation: If you do this exercise in a small group, take turns showing your illustration and explain to the group your best interpretation, including the interpretation of colors selected. Remember that the best person qualified to interpret his or her drawing is the person who drew it. If you do this as a group activity, it's strongly recommended not to interpret other people's work. If you do this by yourself, take a few moments to write about what you have drawn. By articulating your thoughts (verbally or in writing), you make an important link between the conscious and unconscious minds.

Outside Assignments: Once completed, consider hanging your art piece on the fridge or office wall, because often more subtle aspects of interpretation take a while to surface toward conscious recognition.

Art Therapy Color Code

Although there are exceptions, there is a consensus among art therapists (and even psychologists) that regardless of gender, nationality, or ethnic upbringing, each color used in art therapy represents an archetypal meaning. Typically, the color selection, as well as the objects drawn (house, tree, etc.), parallel emotional expressions of one's mental/emotional health. The absence of a color does not mean a lack of something; rather, the colors used express that which the unconscious mind wishes to convey at the time of the drawing. The following list suggests associations between colors and archetypal meanings.

> **Red:** Passionate emotional peaks (from pleasure to pain). It can represent either compassion or anger.
>
> **Orange:** Suggests a life change (big or small, often more positive than negative).
>
> **Yellow:** Represents energy (usually a positive message).
>
> **Green and blue:** Suggest happiness and joy (blue may even mean creativity). These colors also suggest a strong sense or desire of groundedness and stability in your environment.
>
> **Purple or violet:** Suggests a highly spiritual nature, unconditional love.

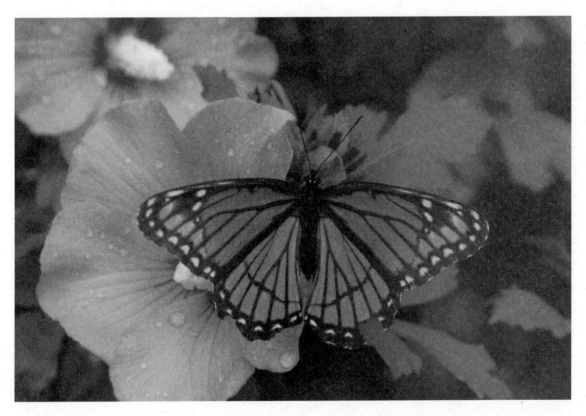

Brown (and earth-tone colors): A sense of groundedness and stability.

Black: Can either represent grief, despair, fear, or a sense of personal empowerment.

White: Can either mean fear, avoidance, cover-up, or hope.

Gray: Typically represents a sense of ambiguity or uncertainty about some issue on which you are working.

Chapter 13

Humor Therapy

EXERCISE **13.1**

In Search of the Proverbial Funny Bone

Laughter is the shortest distance between two people.
Victor Borge

Life is full of absurdities, incongruities, and events that tickle our funny bones. For instance, Chaplin once got third place in a Charlie Chaplin look-alike contest. Since the 1964 day that Norman Cousins checked out of a hospital room into a hotel room across the street and literally laughed his way back to health from a life-threatening disease, the medical world has stood up and taken notice. Humor really *is* good medicine.

Today, there is a whole new scientific discipline, psychoneuroimmunology (PNI), to study the relationship between the mind and the body and the effects each has on the other. It is no secret that negative emotions (e.g., anger, fear, guilt, worry, depression, loneliness) can have a detrimental effect on the body, manifesting as disease and illness. Although there is much to be understood, we now know that, just as negative emotions can have a negative effect on the body, so too positive emotions (e.g., joy, love, hope, and the feelings associated with humor) can have a positive effect on the body by speeding the healing process and promoting well-being.

Humor is a great stress reducer. Humor acts as a coping mechanism to help us deal with life's hardships. It softens (domesticates) the walls of the ego, makes us feel less defensive, unmasks the truth in a comical way, and often gives us a clearer perspective and focus in our everyday lives. Comic relief is used in many stress management programs, hospitals, and work settings. Stress is often associated with negative attitudes that really deflate self-esteem. A preponderance of negative emotions can taint our view of the world, perpetuating the cycle of stress. There has to be a balance. Researchers are now discovering that we need to incorporate positive emotions to achieve balance, and humor is one of the answers.

Although one can turn on the television to catch a few laughs, the greater variety of humor vehicles (books, movies, live comedians, and music) one has access to, the richer the rewards. Sometimes all we have to do is dig through our memory to find a tickler.

1. How would you rate your sense of humor? Do you exercise it often? Do you use it correctly? Offensive humor (sarcasm, racist and sexist humor, practical jokes) can actually promote stress. What are some ways to augment your sense of humor?

2. What is your favorite kind of humor? Parody, slapstick, satire, black humor, nonsense, irony, puns? What type of humor do you fall back on to reduce stress?

3. What would you consider the funniest moment(s) of your life?

4. Are there moments you can recall (from any situation) that are so funny the mere thought puts a grin or secret smile on your face? What are they?

5. In the hit song "My Favorite Things," Julie Andrews sang about a host of things that flooded her mind with joy and brought a smile to her face. What's on your list?

6. Make a list of things to do, places to go, and people to see to lift your spirits when you need it.

_____

_____

_____

_____

_____

_____

_____

_____

_____

_____

_____

_____

_____

_____

_____

_____

EXERCISE **13.2**

Working the Funny Bone

1. It's time to create a new answering machine message. Most likely your answering machine message is the same as everyone else's. Here is an example of a winning voice mail message. See if you can come up with something equally funny:

> Hi, you've reached the home of Bob and Jill. We can't come to the phone right now, because we are doing something we really enjoy. Jill likes doing it up and down. I like doing it sideways. Just as soon as we get done brushing out teeth, we'll call you right back.

Your new voice mail message: _____

_____

_____

_____

2. Humor means "fluid" or "moisture," so let the juice flow! Complete the following sentence by filling in the blank. Combine your talents of creativity and exaggeration to come up with something funny.

You know you're having a bad day when _____

_____

_____

_____

3. You (or a good friend) are new in town and are looking for a new romantic relationship. The problem is shyness, so the solution is a personal ad. Remember that a sense of humor is one of the first things people look for in a mate.

_____

_____

_____

4. You are a vaudevillian songwriter who has been asked to write some new lyrics for the chorus of one of these commonly known songs. Parody a topic (e.g., health care problems, political characters, environmental problems, any news headline).

   a. "Home on the Range"

   b. "Our House"

c. "Cabaret"

d. "My Favorite Things"

e. A rap song

f. Your choice

5. Make a list of your top five movie comedies (with the intention of seeing them again):

a. _____

b. _____

c. _____

d. _____

e. _____

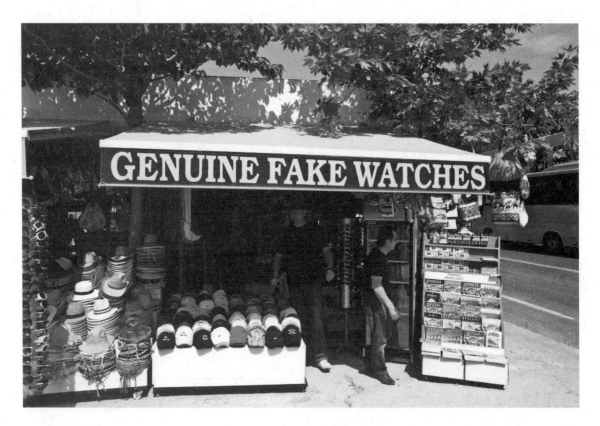

EXERCISE **13.3**

Good Vibrations: Proverbs by First Graders

Part I

A first-grade schoolteacher in Virginia had 25 students in her class. She presented each child in her classroom the first half of a well-known proverb and asked him or her to come up with the remainder of the proverb. It's hard to believe these were actually done by first graders. Their insight may surprise you. While reading, keep in mind that these are first graders, six-year-olds, because the last one is a classic!

Don't change horses . . .	until they stop running.
Strike while the . . .	bug is close.
It's always darkest before . . .	Daylight Saving Time.
Never underestimate the power of . . .	termites.
You can lead a horse to water but . . .	how?
Don't bite the hand that . . .	looks dirty.
No news is . . .	impossible.
A miss is as good as a . . .	Mr.
You can't teach an old dog new . . .	math.
If you lie down with dogs, you'll . . .	stink in the morning.
Love all, trust . . .	me.
The pen is mightier than the . . .	pigs.
An idle mind is . . .	the best way to relax.
Where there's smoke there's . . .	pollution.
Happy the bride who . . .	gets all the presents.
A penny saved is . . .	not much.
Two's company, three's . . .	the Musketeers.
Don't put off till tomorrow what . . .	you put on to go to bed.
Laugh and the whole world laughs with you, cry and . . .	you have to blow your nose.
There are none so blind as . . .	Stevie Wonder.
Children should be seen and not . . .	spanked or grounded.
If at first you don't succeed . . .	get new batteries.
You get out of something only what you . . .	see in the picture on the box.
When the blind lead the blind . . .	get out of the way.

And the *winner* and last one:

Better late than . . .	pregnant.

Part II

Taking a hint from the wisdom of first graders (meaning, think like one), please complete the following proverbs with twenty-first-century pearls of wisdom. Be creative, but most of all, be funny and have fun.

1. Don't get mad . . .   _____

2. A rolling stone . . .   _____

3. A bird in the hand . . .   _____

4. Out of sight . . .   _____

5. Blood is thicker than . . .   _____

6. Fish or . . .   _____

7. Don't throw the baby . . .   _____

8. Easy come . . .   _____

9. Feed a cold . . .   _____

10. Good fences make . . .   _____

11. Here today . . .   _____

12. If you can't beat 'em . . .   _____

13. If you can't stand the heat . . .   _____

14. Once bitten . . .   _____

15. Scratch my back and . . .   _____

16. You made your bed, now . . .   _____

17. Speak softly and . . .   _____

18. It takes a village to . . .   _____

19. The rich get rich and . . .   _____

20. A friend in need is . . .   _____

21. Half a loaf is . . .   _____

22. He who laughs last . . .   _____

23. The grass is always greener . . .   _____

24. Two heads are . . .   _____

25. When in Rome . . .   _____

26. Too many cooks . . .   _____

EXERCISE **13.4**

Making a Tickler Notebook

Consider this! The average child laughs or giggles about three hundred times a day. The typical adult laughs about fifteen times a day. Research reveals that the average hospital patient never laughs at all. This assignment invites you to begin to make a tickler notebook (three-ring notebooks work best) comprising favorite jokes, photographs, images, birthday cards, love letters, Dear Abby columns, poems, or anything else that brings a smile to your face. Keep your tickler notebook on hand so that if you are having a bad day, you can pull it out to help you regain some emotional balance. If you ever find yourself in the hospital for whatever reason, be sure to bring it along so that you can at least get your quota of fifteen laughs a day. Following are two jokes to help you form a critical mass of funny things to include in your notebook.

The New Boss

A company, feeling it is time for a shake-up, hires a new CEO. This new boss is determined to rid the company of all slackers. On a tour of the facilities, the CEO notices a guy leaning on a wall. The room is full of workers, and he wants to let them know he means business. The CEO walks up to the guy and asks, "And how much money do you make a week?" Undaunted, the young fellow looks at him and replies, "I make about $200 a week. Why?"

The CEO hands the guy $1,000 in cash and screams, "Here's a month's pay with benefits, now *get out* and don't come back!"

Surprisingly, the guy takes the cash with a smile, says "Yes sir! Thank you, sir!" and leaves.

Feeling pretty good about his first firing, the CEO looks around the room and asks, "Does anyone want to tell me what that slacker did around here?"

With a sheepish grin, one of the other workers mutters, "Pizza delivery guy from Domino's."

The Bell Curve of Life

At age 4, success is . . . not peeing in your pants.

At age 12, success is . . . having friends.

At age 16, success is . . . having a driver's license.

At age 20, success is . . . having sex.

At age 30, success is . . . having money.

At age 50, success is . . . having money.

At age 60, success is . . . having sex.

At age 70, success is . . . having a driver's license.

At age 75, success is . . . having friends.

At age 80, success is . . . not peeing in your pants!

What are you going to include in your tickler notebook? This assignment includes collecting over twenty items to form a critical mass for your tickler notebook. But don't stop there. Keep gathering jokes, images, birthday cards—*anything* that brings a smile to your face and warms your heart—because you never know when you will need an emotional uplift.

1. _____

2. _____

3. _____

4. _____

5. _____

6. _____

7. _____

8. _____

9. _____

10. _____

11. _____

12. _____

13. _____

14. _____

15. _____

16. _____

17. _____

18. _____

19. _____

20. _____

Creative Problem Solving

EXERCISE **14.1**

The Roles of Creativity

Roger von Oech is right when he states that many hats are worn in the creative process. Reviewing these four specific roles, take some time to examine how you can integrate these creative aspects into your repertoire of skills. If you are like most people, you tend to see yourself as wearing only one of these hats, rather than all four. This is OK when projects or problems require more than one person to contribute their talents. For now, let's assume that you can wear all four hats.

1. **The Explorer.** To help you think outside the box, make a list of ten new places you can explore to find new ideas for any creative project. Next, make a list of five new resources to explore for any creative project.

   a. _____

   b. _____

   c. _____

   d. _____

   e. _____

2. **The Artist.** Inside each and every one of us is an artist begging to play. Make a list of five new ways to engage in the art of play!

   a. _____

   b. _____

   c. _____

   d. _____

   e. _____

3. **The Judge.** How good are your judgmental skills? Are they too good? Are you the kind of person who judges first and asks questions later?

_____

_____

_____

_____

_____

4. **The Warrior.** The warrior is the "legman" in the creative process. A great idea without someone to market it and implement it is not really a great idea. How good are your warrior skills? What can you do to improve them?

_____

_____

_____

EXERCISE **14.2**

Getting the Creative Juices Flowing

Living in our left-brain culture tends to inhibit the creative process. The following exercises are provided to help you whack your way of thinking (from left brain to right brain) so that the creative problem-solving process may become just a bit easier.

I. Create two metaphors or definitions for an optimist and a pessimist.

    a. An optimist is someone who . . .

        1. _____

        2. _____

    b. A pessimist is someone who . . .

        1. _____

        2. _____

II. Describe two things that a cat and a refrigerator have in common.

    _____

    _____

III. Describe the following colors to a person who has been blind from birth.

    a. red _____

    b. white _____

    c. blue _____

    d. green _____

    e. yellow _____

    f. black _____

    g. purple _____

IV. In the following line of letters, cross out six letters so that the remaining letters, without altering their sequence, will spell a familiar English word.

    BSAINXLEATNTEARS _____

V. Create a metaphor for the meaning of life. Finish this sentence:

    Life is like _____

EXERCISE **14.3**

My Creativity Project

This exercise is designed to help inspire you to take some initiative in starting and completing a project that requires some creative license. Initially, this assignment was developed for a holistic health class to fully engage students in the creative process. Many people found this project to be the ticket to a new job. The purpose of this exercise is to challenge you to extend your creative talents to your highest limits. This project involves three aspects:

Part I: First, play the roles of the *explorer*, *artist*, *judge*, and *warrior* respectively, to come up with a very creative idea and then bring it to reality. If you wish, you can use the template in Exercise 14.1 ("The Roles of Creativity") again for this exercise.

Part II: Next, write up the experience, describing what you did (describe your experience in each of the four stages of creativity) and how you accomplished it.

Part III: Finally, explain what you learned from this experience.

The area and magnitude of creativity are entirely up to you. It is suggested, however, that you pick an area that is somewhat familiar (in other words, don't try to build the Brooklyn Bridge if you have never played with Legos), but not one in which you have a five-star command. Challenge yourself! Select a project, which can range anywhere from art, poetry, cooking, composing, photography, designing fashions, writing a screenplay, choreographing a dance, to anything. Start with an interest, passion, or a desire. Build from this a dream. Consult your intuition and then come up with a finished product. Remember that the creative process cannot be rushed or demanded. This assignment will take some time, so plan accordingly.

Make the project manageable. In other words, do not, repeat, do *not* try to build a re-creation of the Eiffel Tower in your backyard or compose the sequel to Handel's *Messiah* in two days. On the other hand, simply putting a new message on your answering machine is not the best way to go either. Make the project a quality job of which you will be proud.

Examples from Previous Students and Workshop Participants

1. Producing a music video presentation.
2. Writing a family/neighborhood cookbook.
3. Producing a YouTube presentation.
4. Creating a holistic cancer treatment plan.
5. Recording/producing a musical CD.
6. Planning a vacation around the world.
7. Designing/planning a rose garden.
8. Writing a nonfiction book proposal.
9. Starting a yoga studio.
10. Organizing a 10K road race for charity.

My Creativity Project: _____

_____

How I Did It (Explain each role of the creative process): _____

_____

_____

_____

_____

_____

_____

_____

_____

_____

_____

What I Learned: _____

_____

_____

_____

_____

_____

_____

_____

EXERCISE **14.4**

Creative Problem Solving

There are many good ways to solve a problem. All you need do is spend some time working at it from different directions until a number of viable solutions surface, and then choose the best one. The following is a time-tested strategic plan for creatively trying to solve problems and come to a sense of resolution.

The Problem: _____

1. **Define or describe the problem.** Please be as specific as you can:

    _____

    _____

    _____

2. **Generate great ideas.** Come up with at least four viable ideas and one zany (x) one to bring out the play factor.

    a. _____

    b. _____

    c. _____

    d. _____

    (x). _____

3. **Select and refine ideas.** Pick the best idea from above and explain why you think this is the best idea.

    _____

    _____

    _____

    _____

    _____

    _____

4. **Implement ideas.** Explain how you will put this idea into action. Make a brief outline—four specific points of your action plan to make this happen.

a. _____

b. _____

c. _____

d. _____

5. **Evaluate and analyze the action plan.** How did the idea work? What ways, if any, are there to improve on this idea should you decide to use it again?

_____

_____

_____

_____

_____

_____

Chapter 15

Communication Skills

EXERCISE **15.1**

What Did You Say?

Conversational skills may not seem like they belong in a stress-management book, but nothing could be further from the truth. Poor conversational skills are often at the root of many stressful relationships. We are engaged in conversation from the moment we wake until the second we lay down our heads and enter the world of dreams. Whether it be family, friends, customers, clients, peers, colleagues, strangers, or even voices on the radio and television, our minds are programmed to listen and respond in conversation virtually every minute of the day.

A proverb states, "The three most important words to a successful relationship are communication, communication, communication." It's true! As social animals we gravitate toward others to engage in conversation. Good communication skills are essential to every aspect of our lives. The elements of conversation are rather complicated because we communicate with more than just words and voices. In fact, more of our communication skills are nonverbal than verbal.

1. How good are your communication skills, both verbal and nonverbal? Are you even aware of the messages you give to others with your clothing style, hair, eye movements, posture, hand gestures, and facial expressions?

2. There is a growing trend among people younger than 30 to prefer text messaging to email and phone calls. Is this your preference? If so, why? Are you aware that some people's e-communication skills are good, but their social (in-person) communication skills are poor? Please explain.

3. Some communication should only be between two people and not for public consumption, yet we are now seeing private conversations become public on Facebook, Twitter, and other social networking sites. Have you ever made a private conversation public? If so, why?

4. What would you say is your body's silent message, that is, without dialogue? Why? Is this the message you wish to convey?

5. Listening skills are as important as the ability to articulate your thoughts and feelings. Yet, most people hear but seldom listen. More often than not, they begin to prepare what they are going to say within seconds of someone beginning to speak or respond. How good are your listening skills? What could you do to improve them?

6. Much research now suggests that men and women have different styles of communication. Have you ever noticed this? For example, have you noticed that when a woman says she'll call you tomorrow, she calls you tomorrow, whereas when a man says he'll call you tomorrow, most likely he will call you in a few days to a week?

7. It has been said that when we speak we are very indirect, not really saying what we mean. We beat around the bush. Do you find that your verbal style is more indirect than direct? Do you tend to give mixed messages? After giving this some thought, can you think of ways to improve your verbal communication skills? Do you need to revise your nonverbal messages? How can you do this?

8. How do your communication styles differ from direct contact to the times when you use your cell phone or text message? Does your cell phone use interfere with your direct personal relationships?

9. Men and women are said to have different communication styles. Although it may be true that men are from Mars and women are from Venus, we are both here on earth, so we have to learn to be bilingual. What differences do you notice talking to the opposite gender? How are these differences magnified in a relationship? Share your thoughts and experiences here.

EXERCISE **15.2**

Communication Skills 101

Gloria Estefan was right when she sang the hit song "Words Get in the Way". They sure do, especially when we are stressed. As a rule, humans tend to be bad communicators when feelings of fear, anger, insecurity, intolerance, or even compassion (not wanting to hurt someone's feelings) cloud what we really wish to say to friends, roommates, spouses, children, and co-workers. Perhaps you've noticed. Below are several statements, questions, or comments that most likely have come out of your mouth on more than one occasion, resulting in miscommunication, hurt feelings, conflict, and perhaps even more stress. Read each comment and then take a moment to come up with a new and diplomatic way to rephrase these statements. Remember the first rule in conflict resolution: Attack issues, not people.

1. You really irritate me.

   _____

2. No, no. Everything is fine.

   _____

3. Oh, we always go there. Let's go here instead.

   _____

4. You want me to do *what*?

   _____

5. Why are you being so difficult?

   _____

6. You do this every time!

   _____

7. Okay, can we just talk about this tomorrow?

   _____

8. I can't take this anymore!

   _____

9. Why can't you do it like this?

_____

10. I need this done by 4:00 P.M. sharp.

_____

11. Because we've always done it this way before!

_____

12. Oh, nothing. It's nothing.

_____

13. I am sick and tired of this!

_____

What expressions do you hear from friends, family, and co-workers that mean something different from what the actual words indicate?

1. _____

2. _____

3. _____

4. _____

Resource Management: Time and Money

EXERCISE **16.1**

My Personal Budget Worksheet

The following is a monthly budget worksheet to help you better see how your personal funds are divided between income and expenses. If your expenses exceed your income, ask yourself what changes can be made to bring these back into balance. Note that personal savings is a necessary expense.

Month:_____

Income

1. Monthly paycheck(s) $ _____
2. Stock dividends $ _____
3. Gifts (e.g., from parents) $ _____
4. Other _____ $ _____
5. Other _____ $ _____
    Total $ _____

Necessary Expenses

1. Rent/Mortgage $ _____
2. Food $ _____
3. Utilities (power/gas) $ _____
4. Phone $ _____
5. Car loan payment $ _____
6. Transportation (gas, car maintenance) $ _____
7. Auto/health insurance $ _____
8. Savings (think of savings as a bill to pay) $ _____

9. Monthly service fees (ISP, athletic club, etc.) $ _____

10. Loan payments (including credit card debt) $ _____

11. Medical and dental $ _____

12. Disposable income (clothes, entertainment, gifts) $ _____

13. Miscellaneous $ _____

14. Other expenses _____ $ _____

15. Other expenses _____ $ _____

16. Other expenses _____ $ _____

     Total $ _____

     Net Gain/Loss: $ _____

Your discretionary income: $ _____/month

EXERCISE **16.2**

Your Relationship with Money

The following are some thought-provoking questions to help you examine your beliefs, attitudes, and behaviors regarding money. There are no wrong answers to these questions. They are merely listed to help you reflect on your fiscal relationships.

1. Do you continually worry about not having enough money?   Yes   No
2. Do you purchase things that you really don't need?   Yes   No
3. Do you spend money on others to make them like you?   Yes   No
4. Do your friends always seem to have things that you wish you had?   Yes   No
5. Do you put 10 percent of your monthly income away in a savings account?   Yes   No
6. Do you know how much it costs you to live each month?   Yes   No
7. Do you typically buy things only to find when you get home that you already have them?   Yes   No
8. Do you eat out more than twice a week?   Yes   No
9. Do you pay to keep things in a storage facility?   Yes   No
10. Are you the kind of person who typically buys on impulse?   Yes   No
11. Do you pay off your credit card each billing cycle?   Yes   No
12. Do you have more than one credit card (e.g., Visa, MasterCard)?   Yes   No
13. As a child, did your parents make you work for an allowance?   Yes   No
14. Look around your house or apartment. Do you really use the items you purchase?   Yes   No
15. Do you spend more than $50 per month on phone calls?   Yes   No
16. When eating out, do you count pennies to determine who owes what?   Yes   No
17. Do you only withdraw money from your bank's ATM?   Yes   No
18. Regardless of how much you make, do you give money to charity?   Yes   No
19. Do you tend to frequently borrow money from friends?   Yes   No
20. Do you frequently buy lottery tickets or gamble in the hopes of winning big bucks?   Yes   No
21. Do you occasionally bounce checks or borrow from your line of credit?   Yes   No
22. Do you use coupons for items you might not otherwise purchase?   Yes   No
23. Do you pay yourself a salary (to be placed in a retirement account)?   Yes   No
24. Do you know your net worth?   Yes   No
25. Do you know your monthly disposable income?   Yes   No

EXERCISE **16.3**

Do You Suffer from Affluenza?

God, all I ask is the chance to prove that money can't buy happiness.
Graffiti at the University of Illinois

There is a disease going around the country that is known to be very infectious. To date there are no known antibiotics to cure it. The disease is affluenza. No one really knows when it started, but it seems to have hit epidemic proportions in the mid-1990s and is still going strong. Originally fueled by a surging economy and an unbridled stock market, affluenza has become a disease to be reckoned with, because no matter the state of economic affairs (good or bad), this disease is now always present.

Affluenza can best be described as an insatiable hunger for the good life, the rich life. It is the consumption of material possessions—hundreds of them. Some people call affluenza an addiction, because unlike a cold or flu, this disease doesn't go away in nine days. The purchase of clothes, CDs, DVDs, cars, and so on serves as a fix to lift one's self-esteem until the novelty has worn off, and then—poof—the process starts all over again. The problem is that buying these items in excess is an attempt to fill a void that can never be filled.

We live in a consumeristic society that rewards this behavior. Listen to people's conversations; within the first five minutes, someone probably mentions something he or she has bought.

Here are some questions to ponder and write about regarding the topic of affluenza:

1. What products have you bought in the past six months? Make a list.
2. Describe in detail how you feel after you make a big purchase in a store.
3. How often do you share the news of this purchase with your friends and family?

_____

_____

_____

_____

_____

_____

_____

_____

EXERCISE **16.4**

Time and Money

It has been said that two of the biggest constraints to leisure are time and money, or the lack thereof. It is no coincidence that these two factors are also two of the leading causes of stress. It is highly unlikely that a check for a million dollars in your mailbox tomorrow would solve your lifelong financial concerns. Neither would an extra hour in the day or an extra day in the week give you more time to get your work done. We are creatures of habit, and chances are that if we had more time and money, we would spend them much as we did before.

Although we may not receive a million dollars or have extra hours in the day, we do have several resources to help us budget these constraints. In the information age of high technology, we are bombarded with interruptions. Time management isn't a luxury; it is a necessity. The keys to good time management include learning to prioritize responsibilities, organize resources, edit the nonessentials, set and evaluate goals, and reward yourself for accomplishments.

Managing money is a different story. It involves separating your wants from your needs, keeping track of income and expenses, and living within your means—not the means of others, as with keeping up with the Joneses. Money management means being disciplined. It means learning to enjoy delayed gratification. It also means finding and enjoying the things in life that are free.

Are time and money, or the lack of each, stressors for you? How does technology become a time robber for you? What is one thing you could start doing right now to manage your time better? Do you have champagne taste on a beer budget? What are some ways that you could gain a better handle on these two constraints to have more leisure and less stress?

_____

_____

_____

_____

_____

_____

_____

_____

_____

EXERCISE **16.5**

The Time-Crunch Questionnaire

Please answer the following questions regarding your time management skills as you are now, not how you would like to be. Add up the numbers you circled and check the questionnaire key to determine your level of time management skills.

1 = rarely   2 = sometimes   3 = often

		Rarely	Sometimes	Often
1.	I tend to procrastinate with projects and responsibilities.	1	2	3
2.	My bedtime varies depending on the workload I have each day.	1	2	3
3.	I am the kind of person who leaves things till the last minute.	1	2	3
4.	I forget to make To Do lists to keep me organized.	1	2	3
5.	I spend more than two hours watching television each night.	1	2	3
6.	I tend to have several projects going on at the same time.	1	2	3
7.	I tend to put work ahead of family and friends.	1	2	3
8.	My life is full of endless interruptions and distractions.	1	2	3
9.	I tend to spend a lot of time on the phone.	1	2	3
10.	Multitasking is my middle name. I am a great multitasker.	1	2	3
11.	My biggest problem with time management is prioritization.	1	2	3
12.	I am a perfectionist when it comes to getting things done.	1	2	3
13.	I never seem to have enough time for my personal life.	1	2	3
14.	I tend to set unrealistic goals to accomplish tasks.	1	2	3
15.	I reward myself before getting things done on time.	1	2	3
16.	I just never have enough hours in the day to get things done.	1	2	3
17.	I can spend untold hours distracted while surfing the Internet.	1	2	3
18.	I tend not to trust others to get things done when I can do them better myself.	1	2	3
19.	If I am completely honest, I tend to be a workaholic.	1	2	3
20.	I have been known to skip meals in order to complete projects.	1	2	3
21.	I will clean my room, garage, or kitchen before I really get to work on projects.	1	2	3
22.	I will often help friends with their work before doing my own.	1	2	3
23.	It's hard to get motivated to get things done.	1	2	3

Questionnaire Key

75–51 points = poor time management skills (time to reevaluate your life skills)

50–26 points = fair time management skills (time to pull in the reins a bit)

0–25 points = excellent time management skills (keep doing what you are doing!)

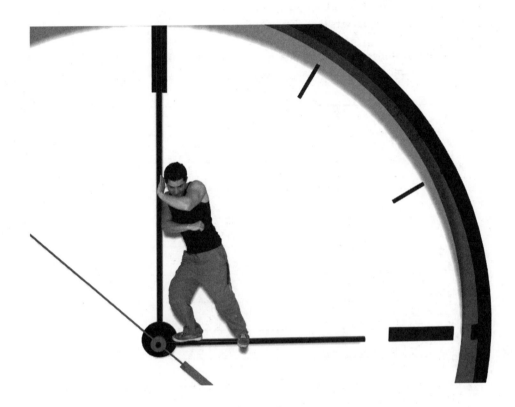

EXERCISE **16.6**

Time Management Idea Exchange

After reading Chapter 16 in *Managing Stress*, please read through the following questions and list the best answers that come to mind.

1. List five reasons people don't manage their time effectively. Which ones apply to your current lifestyle?

   a. _____

   _____

   b. _____

   _____

   c. _____

   _____

   d. _____

   _____

   e. _____

   _____

2. Explain your feelings of stress when your time isn't managed as well as you'd like it to be.

   a. _____

   _____

   b. _____

   _____

   c. _____

   _____

   d. _____

   _____

   e. _____

   _____

3. List the time management techniques that you find most helpful to effectively manage your time and keep you on schedule, and then explain why.

   a. _____

   _____

   b. _____

   _____

   c. _____

   _____

   d. _____

   _____

   e. _____

   _____

4. Think up five new ways to manage your time more effectively (consider including ways to deal with the flood of technology, such as cell phones and email).

   a. _____

   _____

   b. _____

   _____

   c. _____

   _____

   d. _____

   _____

   e. _____

   _____

5. Select one idea from question 3 or 4 that you like and outline the steps you can take to implement this technique.

   a. _____

   _____

   b. _____

   _____

c. _____

_____

d. _____

_____

e. _____

_____

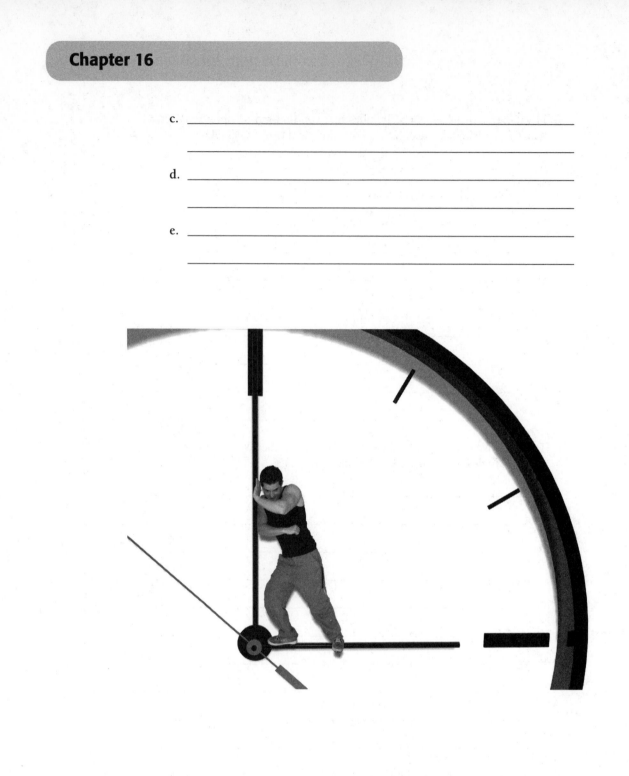

EXERCISE **16.7**

The Importance of Prioritization

The following are two methods of improving your organizational skills for effective prioritization and time management.

To Do List

Date: _____

Write down all the things you need to get done today, with no regard for order.

1.   6.
2.   7.
3.   8.
4.   9.
5.   10.

ABC Rank-Order Method

Direction: In column A, list all the things that you must get done as soon as possible. In column C, list all the things that you would like to do but that are not essential. In column B, put everything else.

A	B	C
_____	_____	_____
_____	_____	_____
_____	_____	_____
_____	_____	_____
_____	_____	_____
_____	_____	_____

Now try organizing your list of things to do in the important-versus-urgent matrix:

Importance

	Low Importance	High Importance
High Urgency	III. A._____ B._____ C._____	I. A._____ B._____ C._____

Urgency

	Low Importance	High Importance
Low Urgency	IV. A._____ B._____ C._____	II. A._____ B._____ C._____

Then begin to work on these tasks in the following order:

I. A._____
    B._____
    C._____
II. A._____
    B._____
    C._____

III. A._____
     B._____
     C._____
IV. A._____
     B._____
     C._____

EXERCISE **16.8**

Time Mapping

The following exercise invites you to chart your day by clearly identifying how each fifteen-minute block of time is actually spent. You can also simply record your daily activities to observe how to best utilize and schedule your time and to see where time robbers are stealing your time in the course of each day.

7:00 A.M. _____

7:15 A.M. _____

7:30 A.M. _____

7:45 A.M. _____

8:00 A.M. _____

8:15 A.M. _____

8:30 A.M. _____

8:45 A.M. _____

9:00 A.M. _____

9:15 A.M. _____

9:30 A.M. _____

9:45 A.M. _____

10:00 A.M. _____

10:15 A.M. _____

10:30 A.M. _____

10:45 A.M. _____

11:00 A.M. _____

11:15 A.M. _____

11:30 A.M. _____

11:45 A.M. _____

12:00 Noon _____

12:15 P.M. _____

12:30 P.M. _____

12:45 P.M. _____

1:00 P.M. _____

1:15 P.M. _____

1:30 P.M. _____

1:45 P.M. _____

2:00 P.M. _____

2:15 P.M. _____

2:30 P.M. _____

2:45 P.M. _____

3:00 P.M. _____

3:15 P.M. _____

3:30 P.M. _____

3:45 P.M. _____

4:00 P.M. _____

4:15 P.M. _____

4:30 P.M. _____

4:45 P.M. _____

5:00 P.M. _____

5:15 P.M. _____

5:30 P.M. _____

5:45 P.M. _____

6:00 P.M. _____

6:15 P.M. _____

6:30 P.M. _____

6:45 P.M. _____

7:00 P.M. _____

7:15 P.M. _____

7:30 P.M. _____

7:45 P.M. _____

8:00 P.M. _____

8:15 P.M. _____

8:30 P.M. _____

8:45 P.M. _____

9:00 P.M. _____

9:15 P.M. _____

9:30 P.M. _____

9:45 P.M. _____

10:00 P.M. _____

After you have written down the events in or plans for the course of your day, what observations can you make from this exercise?

_____

_____

_____

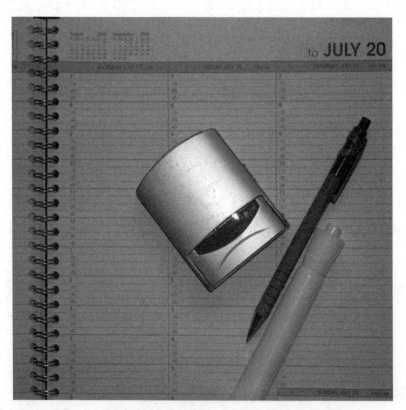

EXERCISE **16.9**

Getting Things Done: The Execution of Tasks

Are you lacking motivation to get some things done? One way to fan the fires of inspiration is to provide some incentives to accomplish big or arduous tasks by giving yourself a reward. Although the real reward is the accomplishment of the deed, a little incentive may be just the thing needed to get it done on time. Remember, not all rewards have to be material possessions. A phone call to a close friend at the end of the day can be as rewarding as a vacation to Tahiti in some cases. Also remember that rewards are meant to decrease stress, not increase it (e.g., food is not always considered a healthy reward).

Goal to Accomplish   *Incentive/Reward*

1. _____   _____

2. _____   _____

3. _____   _____

4. _____   _____

5. _____   _____

6. _____   _____

7. _____   _____

8. _____   _____

9. _____   _____

10. _____   _____

EXERCISE **16.10**

Practicing the Art of Subtraction

Happiness is more a matter of subtraction than addition.
Meister Eckhart

Does your life feel cluttered with too much stuff? Are both your garage and basement filled with stuff that you haven't used (or seen) in years? Do you buy things only to find that when you get home, you now have two of these items? Are there people in your life who are so emotionally needy that when you see them, you want to run and hide? Are there things in your life that at first seemed to simplify things and now seem to be complicating things? If so, you might want to consider engaging in the art of subtraction (also known as "editing your life").

Clutter

Walk through your house or apartment and make a list of five things that fall into the category of personal clutter (this can include equipment, clothes, books, or anything lying on the floor). Once you have made this list, collect the things and consider giving them away to Goodwill or some other charitable organization.

1. _____

2. _____

3. _____

4. _____

5. _____

People

Are there people in your life who take up your time rather than contribute to your quality of life? Take inventory if you have any "friends" who seem to be a drain on your emotional energy. The next question to ask yourself is this: Do you drain other people's energy? Do you give as well as take in your relationships and friendships?

1. _____

2. _____

3. _____

Simplicity Versus Complexity

We tend to bring things into our lives out of both interest and fear. What things are in your life right now that you may have begun out of interest but now are ready to let go? Another way to phrase this question is to ask yourself: What things in your life tend to add complexity rather than simplicity? Once you have identified three things, begin to ask yourself what you can do to subtract these things to bring your life back into balance.

1. _____

2. _____

3. _____

Additional Coping Techniques

EXERCISE **17.1**

Defining Your Support Group

Support groups are vital to the quality and length of our lives. Support groups are composed of friends, colleagues, peers, neighbors, and perhaps most of all, family members. Your support group is made up of those people to whom you feel closest who are there to socialize with, give you a helping hand, or provide a shoulder to cry on when you feel like doing so. The following exercise is designed to help you reinforce the foundations of your support group.

1. Create what you think is the best definition of a friend. A friend is:

   _____

2. Make a list of those people who you feel constitute your support group.

   a. My closest male friends are:

   _____

   b. My closest female friends are:

   _____

   c. The friends I know I can share any problem with at any time include:

   _____

   _____

   d. The friends I can call to go play or go shopping include:

   _____

   _____

e. These friends energize me; they don't drain my energy:

_____

_____

f. Friends on whom I know I can call for a favor at any time include:

_____

_____

g. Friends who are my mentors include:

_____

_____

h. Friends who expand my personal horizons with new ideas or activities are:

_____

_____

3. How has your support group changed over the past five years? Are all of your "friends" on Facebook really part of your support network?

_____

_____

4. Some people in our support groups tend to drain our energy rather than replenish it. Do you have friends like this?

_____

If so, how do you cope with them?

_____

_____

5. What factors in your life detract from your ability to be there for others in your support group?

_____

_____

6. It has often been said that we can never have enough friends. Although this may be true, you cannot spend quality time with everyone, because this weakens the integrity of true friends. What do you do to nurture the connections between you and your friends? In other words, how are you a good friend to others?

_____

_____

7. For a variety of reasons, friends tend to come and go in our lives. New friends can become a collective breath of fresh air in our lives. New friends are harder to make and keep as we age. It helps to continually foster new interests and hobbies. Make a list of three new places where you can begin to meet new people to add as possible members of your support group.

a. _____

b. _____

c. _____

8. Any other comments you wish to share about the topic of friendship?

_____

_____

_____

_____

_____

_____

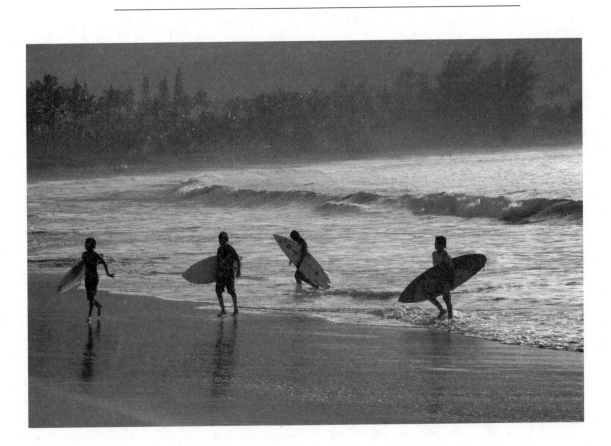

EXERCISE **17.2**

Hobbies and Outside Interests

Here is a question to consider: What would you do for a living if your career didn't exist? Here is another question: If money wasn't a factor in sustaining your desired lifestyle, how would you spend the rest of your life? Hobbies and outside interests provide a sense of balance to the long hours of work that tend to define who we are in this world. The truth is that you are not your job, your career, or even your paycheck. Yet, without claiming some outside interests as a significant part of your life, it becomes easy to see yourself as a passive victim in a rapidly changing world.

1. What are your current outside interests? Name three things or activities in which you partake on a regular (weekly) basis.

    a. _____

    b. _____

    c. _____

2. If you had a hard time coming up with three specific outside interests that qualify as true hobbies, or perhaps you are looking for some new interest to enter your life, consider examples of things you have always wanted to do or to get involved with. What groups or organizations have you wanted to become a member of that can help get you started in this direction?

    a. _____

    b. _____

    c. _____

3. Playing the guitar, knitting a sweater, or making plans to remodel the kitchen are great things to do, but they require time. Making time for hobbies and outside interests requires some discipline. What steps do you take to ensure that you have the time to fulfill the passions of your personal outside interests?

    _____

    _____

    _____

    _____

4. Would you say that your involvement in one or more of your hobbies has a transfer effect on other aspects of your life? If so, how? Please explain:

_____

_____

_____

_____

_____

_____

_____

_____

_____

_____

_____

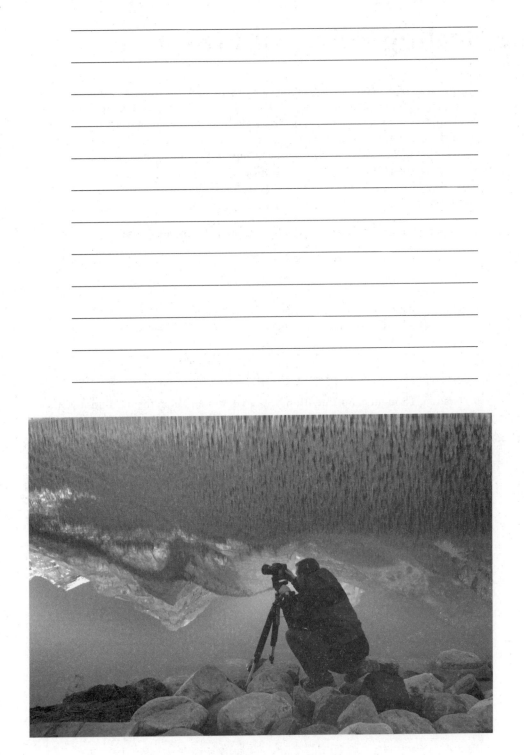

EXERCISE **17.3**

The Healing Power of Prayer

Regardless of one's religious background or lack thereof, prayer is a commonly used coping technique in times of duress. To seek help in times of need is considered a savvy strategy for overcoming problems of any size. Although prayer can be a very personal behavior, we now know that there are certain steps to ensure a clear transmission for divine intercession. Consider using the following outline as a personal template to refine the healing power of your prayers.

Intention: _____

1. **Present Tense:** State your prayerful intention in the present tense.

   _____

   _____

2. **Focused Concentration:** Clear your mind by using the space below to write down any distracting negative thoughts as a means of releasing them.

   _____

   _____

3. **Positive Thoughts and Intentions:** State your intention in the most positive way.

   _____

   _____

4. **Emotional Vibration:** Call to mind the most favorable emotions you can feel. If it helps, write down the experience and feeling to help recreate this feeling now.

   _____

   _____

5. **Detached Outcomes:** Below, write any fears, anxieties, or desires that need to be released to make the prayer fly.

   _____

   _____

6. **Attitude of Gratitude:** Take a moment to write a few words of thanks here for that for which you are grateful.

   _____

   _____

   _____

EXERCISE **17.4**

Friends in Need

And let there be no purpose in friendship, save the deepening of the spirit.
Kahlil Gibran, *The Prophet*

What is a friend? Perhaps it's someone with whom to share precious moments of your life. Perhaps a friend is a person to whom we confide our innermost thoughts and feelings. Maybe a friend is someone just to be there when we need a helping hand or a comforting hug. Friends are all this and more.

Human beings are social by nature. Although times of being alone can serve as a great way to energize the soul, it is to our advantage to balance solitude with interactions. We need exchanges with people to whom we feel close, our network of friends and family.

Some interesting findings have emerged from research investigating the health and longevity of the world's oldest living citizens. We now know that involvement with friends, who make up our social support group, is as important to our health as regular exercise, proper nutrition, and sleep. In troubled times our friends can help buffer or neutralize the stress and tension we feel and serve as an effective means to cope with stress.

As we grow and mature in our own lives, so do the relationships with our friends. The bonds we have with some people continually strengthen over time and distance, whereas others seem to fray or fade. We often attract people into our lives with similar interests and ambitions. In some cases, our closest friends can seem more like family than our brothers and sisters. In every case, friendships, like houseplants and pets, need attention and nurturing. Every now and then, it is a good idea to take a moment to evaluate our friendships to see whether they are truly fulfilling our needs. This inventory of friends can let us know if we have outgrown, or grown apart from, some people, and why. It can also make us aware of the qualities that constitute a good, close, or best friend, and the difference between a good friend and an acquaintance. We also need to evaluate whether we are making an equal contribution to each relationship. Here are some questions to help you with this assessment.

1. How would you best define the word *friend?* What does being a friend mean to you?

2. What is it that draws a person into your life to become a friend?

3. Make a list of all your current friends. Are any members of your family in this group? How has this list changed over the past five years?

4. How would you evaluate your current circle of friends? Do you have several acquaintances that you call friends?

5. Does your support group consist of people in different social circles, or is yours a closed circle of friends? Why would friends in different circles be of value?

6. What keeps your bonds of friendship strong, and what tends to let some friendships fade away?

7. Are there any additional comments you wish to add here?

223

EXERCISE **17.5**

Sweet Forgiveness

You cannot shake hands with a clenched fist.
Indira Gandhi

Every act of forgiveness is an act of unconditional love. If unresolved anger is a toxin to the spirit, then forgiveness is the antidote. Where anger is a roadblock, forgiveness is a ladder to climb above and transcend the experience. For forgiveness to be complete and unconditional, you must be willing to let go of all feelings of anger, resentment, and animosity. Sweet forgiveness cannot hold any taste of bitterness, because these feelings are mutually exclusive. Victimization is a common feeling when one encounters stressors in the form of another person's behaviors. When we sense that our human rights have been violated, feelings of rage can quickly turn into feelings of resentment. Left unresolved, these toxic thoughts can taint the way we treat others and ourselves.

Forgiving those who we feel have wronged us is not an easy task. Often it's a process, and at times, a very long process at that. Yet turning the other cheek does not mean you have to let people walk all over you. Forgiveness is not a surrender of your self-esteem, nor is it a compromise of your integrity. When you can truly forgive the behavior of those by whom you feel violated, you let go of the feelings of control and become free to move on with your life. Resentment and grudges can become roadblocks on the human path. Forgiveness turns a hardened heart into an open passageway to progress on life's journey. Think for a moment of someone who might have violated your humanness. Is it time to let go of some toxic thoughts and initiate a sense of forgiveness?

To begin this journal entry, write the name of that person or those persons toward whom you feel some level of resentment. Beside each name write down what action or behavior it was that offended you and why you feel so violated. What feelings arise in you when you see this person or even hear his or her name? Next, make a note of how long you have felt this way toward this person. Finally, search your soul for a way to forgive the people on your list, even if it means just acknowledging their human spirit. Then practice the act of forgiveness as best you can, and let the feelings of resentment go.

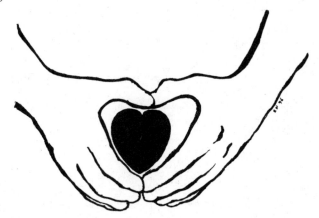

Diaphragmatic Breathing

EXERCISE **18.1**

Dolphin Breath Meditation

Meditation Script

Introduction

Breathing is, perhaps, the most common way to promote relaxation. Taking a few moments to focus on your breathing, to the exclusion of all other thoughts, helps to calm mind, body, and spirit. By focusing solely on your breathing, you allow distracting thoughts to leave the conscious mind. In essence, clearing the mind of thoughts is very similar to deleting unwanted emails, thus allowing more room to concentrate on what is really important in your life, that which really deserves attention.

Script

In a normal resting state, the average person breathes about fourteen to sixteen breath cycles per minute. Under stress, this can increase to nearly thirty breath cycles per minute. Yet in a deep relaxed state, it is not uncommon to have as few as four to six breath cycles in this same time period. The breathing style that produces the greatest relaxation response is that which allows the stomach to expand, rather than the upper chest (this is actually how you breathe when you are comfortably asleep). Take a few moments to breathe, specifically focusing your attention on your abdominal area. And, if any distracting thoughts come to your attention, simply allow these to fade away as you exhale.

Sometimes, combining visualization with breathing can augment the relaxation response. The dolphin breath meditation is one such visualization. Imagine if you will that, like a dolphin, you have a hole in the crown of your head with which to breathe. Although you will still breathe through your nose or mouth, imagine that you are now taking in slow, deep breaths through the opening at the top of your head.

As you do this, feel the air or energy come in through the top of your head, down past your neck and shoulders, and reside momentarily at the base of your spine.

Then, when you feel ready, very slowly exhale, allowing the air to move back out through the dolphin spout, the opening situated at the top of your head. As you slowly exhale, feel a deep sense of inner peace reside throughout your body.

Once again, using all your concentration, focus your attention on the opening at the top of your head. Now, slowly breathe air in through this opening—comfortably slow, comfortably deep. As you inhale, feel the air move down into your lungs, yet allow it to continue further down, deep into your abdominal region. When you feel ready, slowly exhale, allowing the air to move comfortably from your abdominal region up through the top of your head.

Now, take three slow, deep dolphin breaths, and each time you exhale, feel a deep sense of relaxation throughout your body.

1. (Pause) . . . Inhale . . . five to ten seconds . . . Exhale
2. (Pause) . . . Inhale . . . five to ten seconds . . . Exhale
3. (Pause) . . . Inhale . . . five to ten seconds . . . Exhale

Just as you imagined a hole in the top of your head, now imagine that in the sole of each foot there is also a hole through which you can breathe. As you create this image, take a slow, deep breath and through your mind's eye visualize air coming in through the soles of each foot. Visualize the air moving in from your feet, up through your legs, past your knees and waist, to where it resides in your abdominal region. When you feel ready, begin to exhale slowly and allow the air to move back out the way it came, out through the soles of your feet.

Using all your concentration, again focus your attention on the openings at the bottom of your feet and once again breathe in air through these openings, comfortably slow, comfortably deep. As before, feel the air move up your legs and into your abdominal region as your lungs fill with air. Then, when you feel ready, exhale, allowing the air to move slowly from your abdominal region, back through your legs and out the soles of your feet.

Once again, please take three slow, deep breaths, this time through the soles of your feet; and each time you exhale, feel a deep sense of relaxation all throughout your body.

1. (Pause) . . . Inhale . . . five to ten seconds . . . Exhale
2. (Pause) . . . Inhale . . . five to ten seconds . . . Exhale
3. (Pause) . . . Inhale . . . five to ten seconds . . . Exhale

Now, with your concentration skills fully attentive, with your mind focused on the openings of *both* the top of your head and the soles of your feet, use your imagination to inhale air through both head and feet. As you do this, slowly allow the passage of air entering from both head and feet to move toward the center of your body, where it resides in the abdominal region until you exhale. Then, when you feel ready, slowly exhale and direct the air that came in through the top of your head to exit through the dolphin hole, while at the same time directing the air that entered through the soles of your feet to leave from that point of entry. Once you have tried this, repeat this combined breath three times, and with each exhalation, notice how relaxed your body feels.

1. (Pause) . . . Inhale . . . five to ten seconds . . . Exhale
2. (Pause) . . . Inhale . . . five to ten seconds . . . Exhale
3. (Pause) . . . Inhale . . . five to ten seconds . . . Exhale

When you're done, allow this image to fade from your mind, but retain the sense of deep relaxation this experience has instilled throughout your mind, body, and spirit. Then take one final slow, deep breath, feeling the air come into your nose or mouth, down into your lungs, and allow your stomach to extend out and then deflate as you begin to exhale. Again, feel a deep sense of calm as you exhale.

When you feel ready, allow your eyes to slowly open to a soft gaze in front of you, and bring your awareness back to the room where you now find yourself. As you bring yourself back to the awareness of the room you are now in, you feel fully energized, recharged, revitalized, and ready to accomplish whatever tasks await you ahead.

Thoughts and Experiences

_____

_____

_____

_____

_____

_____

_____

_____

_____

_____

_____

_____

_____

Meditation

Meditation. . . . It's not what you think!
—Anonymous

EXERCISE **19.1**

Too Much Information

If no one has officially said this to you yet, then you are overdue to hear these words: "Welcome to the information age!" Satellite television, cable television, the Internet, cell phones, and embedded computer chips are just a few things that inundate us with a tsunami of information. As if this weren't enough, there are more things looming on the horizon, all of which are begging for our attention. If you are like most people today, most likely you are drowning in information. There is even a new name for this: information stress.

Although we take in information through all of our five senses, over 80 percent of all the information we take in is received through the senses of sight and sound. Well before the term "information age" was coined, it was very easy to experience sensory overload from too much information taken from the eyes and ears, such as from watching too much television to pulling an all-nighter to cram for an exam. The consequence of sensory overload is becoming numb to it all and walking around like a zombie. It's no stretch to say there are people who fit this description.

Living in the information age, discernment is essential. Discernment means being able to distinguish truth from non-truth. Perhaps more accurately, it means discerning news from marketing, news from entertainment, and truth from hype and spin.

There is a solution to information overload. It is a practice called meditation: cleaning the mind of all the clutter and useless information that bombards your attention span.

1. List five ways to successfully decrease the quantity of information with which you are barraged every day.

   a. Turn off TV (limit time)

   b. Use commute time as "QUIET TIME"

   c. Read (but use an actual Book - Ø tablet)

   d. Set time limit on computer

   e. No TV in bedroom (QUIET ZONE)

2. People tend to mirror behavior, often not even knowing that they do this. In terms of too much information, or TMI, people who take in too much information often talk to their friends and share too much information (e.g., how much they make, how many times they have sex per week, or how often they clean their bathroom). There is a_real art to sharing information without revealing everything. As a rule, people who share too much information about themselves have acceptance problems. Are you the kind of person who volunteers too much information? If so, what can you do to filter out the less important facts and perceptions and still get your point across?

Not really, I am not as private as my mom was + sister is; however there is value to sharing when you feel you are the only one going thru something - isolation is Ø good; it can be helpful to learn from someone else how they deal with stress.

3. See if you can come up with a handful of ways to bring balance back into your life by taking time to quiet your mind and explain them here.

① Again: get back into Church -
② When adding something to my "to do" list, take away something
③ Read for pleasure
④ Date night w/ hubby
⑤ " " " w/ kids

EXERCISE **19.2**

Focus!

Are you one of the millions of Americans diagnosed as having attention deficit disorder (ADD)? If you are, you are in good company. It seems nearly everyone has a shortened attention span these days. It may be hard to imagine, but not long ago, television commercials were thirty to sixty seconds long. Then came the invention of the remote control. Now commercial sponsors duel with your attention span in the hopes they can get their message across before your thumb makes a move. Take a look at the time spent on each scene, and you will notice that the camera is almost always moving. This keeps your attention by triggering the stress response. Add to the equation the introduction of video games and it would appear that technology has played a very big role in undermining the national attention span. But that is not all. There are a host of chemical substances we ingest (e.g., aspartame and MSG), often without knowing, that also affect our conscious thought process.

In his book *Excitotoxins*, author Russell Blaylock describes various food substances that greatly affect brain function. The two most commonly ingested excitotoxins are aspartame (more commonly known as NutraSweet and Equal) and MSG (monosodium glutamate). These two substances, as well as a host of artificial colors, flavors, and preservatives, have a serious effect on cognitive function. Aspartame and MSG cross the blood-brain barrier.

Tibetan sages suggest that everyone, at some level, has ADD. If you have an ego, then join the club. More than likely, the ability to focus your attention is based on the coming together of a great many factors. Here is a chance to look at your health behaviors and see whether there are things you do that contribute to a poor attention span. Here is a challenge: Come up with ten behaviors in which you partake that you feel decrease your mental focus. Explain each one.

_____

_____

_____

_____

_____

_____

_____

_____

_____

EXERCISE **19.3**

Bridging the Hemispheres of Thought

In 1956 a researcher named Roger Sperry conducted some experiments on a handful of patients with grand mal epileptic seizures. In the procedure he created, he cut the *corpus callosum*, the bridge of neural fibers that connects the right and left hemispheres of the brain. Not only did the operation reduce the number and intensity of the grand mal seizures, but it also soon gave credence to a whole new concept of how the mind, through the brain, processes information. Roger Sperry's research led to a Nobel Prize in medicine and to the household expressions *right-brain thinking* and *left-brain thinking*.

Left-brain thinking skills are associated with judgment, analysis, mathematical and verbal acuity, linear thought progression, and time consciousness; right-brain functioning is associated with global thinking, holistic thinking, imagination, humor, emotionality, spatial orientation, receptivity, and intuition.

Western culture grooms and rewards left-brain thinking. It is fair to say that judgmental thinking is one of our predominant traits. Although it is true that Western culture is left-brain dominant in thinking skills, the truth of the matter is that to be dominant in one style of thinking is actually considered lopsided and imbalanced.

1. How would you describe your dominant thinking style? Would you say that your left brain or right brain dominates?

2. If you were to make a guess or assumption as to why your thinking skills gravitate toward one direction or the other, what would be your explanation?

3. One of the basic themes of wellness is balance—in this case, balance of the right-brain and left-brain functions. Based on your answer to the first question, what are your dominant thinking skills and your nondominant thinking skills? What are some ways you can balance your patterns by bridging between the right and left hemispheres of your brain?

_____

_____

_____

_____

_____

_____

_____

EXERCISE **19.4**

Celestial Heavens Meditation

Meditation Script

Imagine that this evening is a warm summer night—neither hot, nor humid, but comfortably warm. You step outside the back door and feel a slight breeze in the air, and it feels really nice against your face.

The sun has set, but it's still somewhat light. You look up in the sky and it is full of clouds—big, billowy clouds. The sun's last rays light up the clouds on the western horizon, and this light turns the gray clouds pink and orange for a few lingering moments. Tonight, the sky looks so inviting.

As you stand at the back door, you think to yourself how nice it would be to grab a blanket and lie under the stars for a few hours. Then you think to yourself, "Hey, why not?" So you go back inside, grab a blanket, perhaps even a pillow, and then head back outside again.

After meandering a ways, you find a nice comfortable spot, far away from any city lights—your own private place to lie down and relax. You spread the blanket out and then lie down. Notice how good it feels to connect with the earth. Again you feel the summer breeze upon your face, and it feels good too.

From the time you first looked outside tonight to this very moment, you noticed that the sky has filled with more clouds, but you also notice that the winds have picked up and they quickly move the clouds from west to east across the night sky. Every now and then, you see what looks like an evening star peeking through the clouds. You look closely, but your mind begins to wander, and the star hides again.

Metaphorically speaking, clouds are like thoughts in your mind, and tonight these clouds represent the multitude of thoughts racing through your mind. The purpose of this meditation, this time looking up in the sky, is to clear your mind of excess thoughts; persistent, nagging thoughts; and random thoughts so that your mind becomes as clear as the clearest night sky.

Specifically, these clouds overhead, these big, billowy clouds, are symbolic of any thoughts, issues, problems, or conflicts that you are facing in your life right now. As you see a cloud overhead, label it with whatever thought that comes to mind, take a nice deep breath, and as you exhale, let it go as you watch the wind carry the cloud away. In doing so, you allow yourself to detach from this thought or concern long enough to gain a better sense of clarity. Once again, take a nice, slow, deep breath and allow each cloud above to slowly disappear from view over the eastern horizon.

Every now and then you glimpse a star twinkling through the clouds. The first stars to appear in the night sky are typically our neighboring planets. Take a moment to focus on a star, but then notice it is quickly covered up as another cloud comes into view. As you see this next cloud come into view, bring to mind another stressor—some frustration or anxiety—label the cloud with it, and then watch it move across the horizon, fading from view. Once again, take a nice slow, deep breath and allow this cloud and the thought it represents to slowly disappear from view over the eastern horizon.

Every cloud that comes into view represents some problem or issue, but tonight, the cool wind acts like a broom to sweep away all these thoughts and concerns, leaving your mind clear and still. Allow the wind to carry your thoughts and concerns away off to the horizon and beyond. Notice that as these clouds begin to move away from your field of vision, your body and mind become more and more relaxed. Once again, take a nice, slow, deep breath and allow the cloud overhead to slowly disappear from view over the eastern horizon.

Concentrate and look up in the sky. Tonight, and every night, the sky serves as a metaphor of your mind. As you gaze up to the heavens, you notice that above the layer of thick, billowy clouds, there is a very thin layer of cloud as well, so thin that you can faintly see the brightest stars shine through. This layer of clouds is also being pushed by the wind from west to east, and it moves high above your head. This layer of cloud represents any lingering thoughts, any random thoughts, or perhaps any excess energy that distracts your attention away from the celestial sea that it veils. Take a nice, deep, slow breath and allow this thin layer of clouds to slowly disappear over the horizon.

Above you now the sky is clear, and the stars are so near you can practically reach out and touch them. As you gaze upward, you see in front of you the Milky Way stretched thick and wide across the sky, as if someone took a paintbrush across the sky. As you focus on the stars, you begin to recognize familiar constellations: the Big Dipper, Orion, or perhaps the Pleiades.

Stars in the night sky are points of light that convey brilliance and wisdom. Take a moment to pick one star and focus your entire awareness on it. Once again, take a nice, deep, slow breath, and as you exhale, feel a sense of deep peace throughout your mind and body, as deep as the celestial sky. Take one more slow, deep breath, and this time as you exhale, allow your eyes to wander until they find another star to focus on. Again feel a deep sense of inner peace.

When you feel ready, close your eyes to this image and bring your awareness back to your body. Once again take a nice, slow, deep breath and feel a profound sense of relaxation throughout your mind and body.

Imagine yourself sitting up on the blanket, then standing up and picking up the blanket and turning toward the direction of home. Soon you find yourself back on your back porch and then, in the blink of an eye, you are lying comfortably on your bed. Become aware of how relaxed you are, yet how energized you feel, refreshed and renewed.

When you feel ready, slowly open your eyes to a soft gaze in front of you, and bring yourself back to the awareness of the room you are now in.

Remind yourself that although you feel relaxed, you do not feel sleepy or tired. In fact, you feel re-energized and renewed. On your next breath as you exhale, think to yourself the phrase "I am re-energized and renewed and inspired to continue whatever projects await me today."

Thoughts and Experiences

_____

_____

_____

_____

_____

_____

_____

_____

_____

_____

_____

_____

_____

_____

_____

_____

_____

_____

_____

_____

_____

_____

_____

_____

_____

Hatha Yoga

EXERCISE **20.1**

Hatha Yoga Revisited

Hatha yoga, as a mind-body exercise, has been around for generations. Its popularity has increased dramatically over the past decade, making hatha yoga more popular to-day than cardiovascular exercise in many parts of the country. More than just basic stretching, Hatha yoga is a practice of achieving balance within the body's structure as well as a union of mind, body, and spirit. This worksheet serves as a means to refresh your memory regarding some of the basics of hatha yoga as well as to have you artic-ulate how this means of relaxation—whether it was a one-time experience or a regular part of your daily routine—has felt for you personally.

Hatha Yoga Review

Please answer the following in a sentence or two.

1. What does the word *hatha* mean?

   _____

2. What does the word *yoga* mean?

   _____

3. List two other types or styles of yoga.

   _____

4. What is the "Salute to the Sun"?

   _____

5. What is the "pranayama"?

   _____

6. What is the "Shavasana"?

   _____

Mind-Body Processing

1. Describe in a few sentences what your body feels like right after a hatha yoga session.

   _____

2. In your own words, what do you feel is the essence of hatha yoga?

   _____

3. What has hatha yoga done for you mentally, physically, and emotionally?

   _____

4. How does hatha yoga help alleviate pain or chronic pain?

   _____

5. Please share any other comments regarding hatha yoga at this time here:

   _____

   _____

   _____

   _____

   _____

   _____

   _____

   _____

   _____

   _____

   _____

   _____

   _____

   _____

Mental Imagery and Visualization

EXERCISE **21.1**

I Have a Vision: The Art of Visualization

A popular song back in the 1960s had a line that went like this: "Thinking is the best way to travel." In many ways this is true. The mind has an incredible ability to project itself to many places—some places the body might have been to, some only the mind visits in dreams. Traveling on the thoughts generated by the mind, we can go anywhere. No ticket or baggage is required, only a desire and your imagination.

If you had the ability to project yourself anywhere to relax for an hour or so, where would you go? This journal theme invites you to plan five mental mini-vacations and then use the powers of your imagination to take you there.

Visualization can also be used to heal the body by using your imagination to create a vision of restored health of a specific organ or region of your body. In fact, visualization is one of the leading techniques in mind-body medicine.

The purpose of this exercise, then, is to sharpen your imagination and relaxation skills so that when you recognize your need to unwind you can escape, if only momentarily, to a place that gives you peace of mind. When drafting these images, give as much detail as possible so you can not only see them in your mind's eye, but actually feel yourself there through all five senses.

What are some healing visualizations you can use to restore yourself to health?

The CD that accompanies the text, *Managing Stress*, has two guided mental imagery tracks: (1) A Mountain Lake and (2) Rainbow Meditation. Listen to each of these and write your impressions of each in the following space.

_____

_____

_____

_____

EXERCISE **21.2**

Three Short Guided Visualizations

A Point of Light in Space

This guided imagery is called a point of light in space. As with all types of guided imagery, please adapt and embellish all suggestions you hear to best promote a sense of rest and relaxation. To begin . . . .

Close your eyes and begin to focus on your breathing. Feel the air come into your nose or mouth, down into your lungs, and as you inhale, feel your stomach area extend out comfortably. Then when you begin to exhale, feel a deep sense of relaxation, for there is no work, no effort, as you release the air from your lungs. This is the most relaxed part of breathing. The exhalation phase of the breath cycle requires no work, no effort—it happens all by itself. Please repeat this cycle of comfortably deep breathing two more times. Inhale (pause five seconds). Exhale. Inhale (pause five seconds). Exhale.

Now, with your mind's eye, imagine a vast area of dark empty space in front of you. As you look at this dark empty space, off in the distance you see a small point of light: a brilliant, golden-white light. Allow your thoughts to slowly bring this point of light closer to you. Think to yourself of the stillness that surrounds the light. The stillness represents the quiet solitude that the mind craves after a busy day of sensory overload. The point of light represents only that which is essential to focus on for your higher good. All other thoughts are unimportant at this time. Once again, focus on the small point of light. Although this point of light is small, it's bright and vibrant. This light is a symbolic representation of yourself—yourself at complete homeostasis.

As you focus on this point of light, take a slow, comfortable, deep breath—as slow and comfortably deep as you can. As you exhale, place all of your attention, all of your concentration, on this point of light. If your mind should happen to wander, and most likely it will, simply direct all thoughts back to this point of light in a calm sea of still darkness.

As you focus on this point of light, think to yourself that in the course of a busy day you are constantly being bombarded with sensory stimulation and an abundance of information. Although the mind seeks stimulation, the mind also craves time to unwind and relax. Balance is essential. While it may be impossible to have no thoughts in your mind, it is possible to focus solely on just one thought. Right now, the only thought you need to focus on is this beautiful point of light. As you focus on this single point of brilliant light, take one more slow, deep breath. As you exhale, feel whatever tensions or excess energy you carry in your mind dissipate, thus allowing for a deeper sense of relaxation of mind, body, and spirit.

Take one more slow, deep breath, and this time as you exhale, slowly allow this image of the brilliant point of light to fade from your mind's eye, yet retain the deep sense of relaxation and calm it has instilled. And as you do this, begin to place all of your attention on your breathing. Inhale and as you do, feel your stomach begin to extend, then slowly come back in as you exhale. In this exhalation process, become aware of a deep sense of complete relaxation.

245

Although you feel relaxed, you don't feel sleepy or tired. You feel refreshed and renewed. As you become aware of this energizing sensation, begin to open your eyes to a soft gaze in front of you and slowly bring yourself back to the awareness of the room you are now in, feeling refreshed and renewed.

Gentle Falling Snow

Picture this: You are sitting by a large picture window in a warm log cabin on a brisk winter's day. You have the entire place to yourself, and the solitude feels invigorating. There is a log fire in the wood stove radiating abundant heat. Both the sounds of crackling wood and the scent of pine arouse your senses and for a moment, you close your eyes and take a slow, deep breath, a sigh that refreshes. As you exhale, you feel a wonderful sense of relaxation permeate your entire body from head to toe, and it feels great. Consciously, you take another slow, deep breath in through your nose. As you exhale through your mouth, you become aware of the glorious stillness that surrounds you in this cabin.

From where you are seated, look out the window, and as you do, you see falling snow, snow that falls gently to the ground in large flakes. Everything outside is covered in white fluffy snow: the ground, the pine trees, the aspens—in fact, all the trees for as far as you can see are covered in snow. As you look closely at the snowflakes descending from on high toward the ground, you sense a calmness both indoors and outdoors. Other than snow falling, everything is still. Everything is quiet. This stillness you observe is a reflection of the tranquility you feel within yourself.

This stillness is so inviting that you slowly move off the couch and stand up. As you walk toward the cabin door, you put on your warm winter coat, hat, and gloves. Then, slowly you open the door and simply stand in the doorframe to observe the endless dance of millions of snowflakes floating gently—almost in slow motion—from the sky down to the snow-covered ground.

Listen closely. What do you hear? The sound of snowflakes is so soft, so gentle, that the sound is barely audible. Your ability to focus on this sound to the exclusion of all other thoughts sets your mind at ease, like a broom that gently sweeps the floor of any remnants needing to be cleaned. The snow-covered ground is a symbol of your mind: clean, clear, and still. Take a slow, deep breath of this clean, fresh air and feel a deeper sense of calmness throughout your entire body.

As you step back inside and close the door, you kick off your shoes, take off this jacket, hat, and gloves, and return to the couch by the picture window.

As you close your eyes to focus on the sounds of stillness, take one final slow, deep breath and bring that stillness into the center of your heart space.

Now, slowly allow this image to fade from your mind's eye, but retain the sense of tranquility it inspired. Make yourself aware of your surroundings: the room, the building, the time of day, and perhaps what you will do after this relaxation session. Although you feel relaxed, you don't feel tired. You feel rested and rejuvenated. Begin to make yourself aware of your body. Stretch your arms and shoulders. When you feel ready, open your eyes to a soft gaze in front of you, and as you do, retain this sense of calm comfort throughout your mind, body, and spirit all day long.

A Walk on a Secluded Beach

The beach, from the warm turquoise waters of the ocean to the cool, gentle breezes and warm sand, has served humanity for thousands of years as a metaphor for cleansing the mind and relaxing the body. Sitting or walking along a deserted beach and focusing on the gentle rhythm of the ocean surf serve a primal desire for relaxation. It is this image that we wish to re-create in the mind's eye for the same purpose right now.

The time of day is moments before sunrise, or if you wish, sunset. The temperature is comfortably warm, yet there is a gentle breeze in the air. The sky contains a few clouds, but only enough to enhance the spectacle of reflecting the sun's rays in concert with the rotation of the earth. While there may be birds off in the distance, you notice that the only sounds you hear are those of the ocean waves in perfect rhythm with your relaxed breathing: inhalation and exhalation.

As you stop for a moment and look out to the horizon, the vastness of all you see in front of you shrinks any and all problems, concerns, and issues you may have at this time to their proper proportion. The immensity, as well as the beauty, of the view you hold in your eyes is exhilarating. Stop for a moment and take a comfortably slow, deep breath. Just as the ocean's waves clean the shoreline, so too does each exhalation cleanse your mind and body of any thoughts, attitudes, perceptions, beliefs, and feelings that, at one time, may have served you but now only hold you back. Using the ocean surf as a metaphor for peace and relaxation, breathe several times for the next several minutes in rhythm with the ocean's tide to instill a deep sense of peace and relaxation in both your mind and your body.

Inhale . . . (pause five to ten seconds) . . . Exhale

Inhale . . . (pause five to ten seconds) . . . Exhale

Inhale . . . (pause five to ten seconds) . . . Exhale

Inhale . . . (pause five to ten seconds) . . . Exhale

And one more time: Inhale . . . (pause five seconds) . . . Exhale.

As you exhale, take a moment to look down in the sand. As you do, you notice a seashell that catches your attention. You bend down to pick it up and feel the soft texture of the repeated eons of surf on each side of this shell. With a smile of recognition that we too will become soft to the touch with the repeated surf of time, you place this shell in your pocket as a reminder of your own journey of personal growth.

Now, slowly allow this image to fade from your mind, but retain all sensations of relaxation. As you do this, return all thoughts to your breathing each breath comfortably calm and relaxed.

Make yourself aware of your surroundings. Remember, although you feel relaxed, you don't feel tired or sleepy. You feel rested and rejuvenated. Begin to make yourself aware of your body. Stretch your arms and shoulders. When you feel ready, open your eyes to a soft gaze in front of you and bring yourself back to awareness of your current surroundings.

Thoughts and Experiences

_____

_____

_____

_____

Chapter 22

Music Therapy

EXERCISE **22.1**

Good Vibrations: From Sound to Music

The following are some exercises to engage more fully in the practice of music therapy.

1. **Make (mix) your own music playlist Rx.** Today's technology makes it very easy for you to compile your favorite instrumental songs. Here is a suggestion: Make a playlist of 12 to 16 of your favorite instrumental pieces and write them down. Be sure to include not only a variety of styles (e.g., classical, new age, jazz) but also a variety of instrumentation (e.g., piano, guitar, violin, cello). Then burn it onto a CD. Consider burning a few extra copies: one for the car when you get stuck in traffic, one for the office when things there go haywire, and one for home to listen to late at night to help you unwind.

2. **Finding the lost chord.** Not everyone is blessed with a great singing voice, but you don't have to have one to do this exercise. Remind yourself of the location of the chakras, find a nice quiet place (preferably where no one will hear you) and simply voice the word *Om* (Ohhmmmmmmmmmmmmm). Carry the note for about thirty seconds, starting with the root chakra, then taking a slight pause, and then moving up through the line of chakras. (This may feel really weird, but that's why you have closed the door.) Try repeating this cycle about three to four times. You can also find CDs with the om chant and merely sing along. (Synchronicity has an *Om* CD [1.800.926.2033], as does Jonathan Goldman, whose CD is called *Chakra Chants*.)

    A variation of this exercise is to sing the scale (do, re, mi, fa, sol, la, ti, do), starting with the lowest note and continuing up the scale through each of the seven notes (seven notes—seven chakras).

3. **Music and visualization.** For this exercise, find a CD or playlist with instrumental music. Those listed as New Age work the best (two suggestions: John Serrie's *And the Stars Go With You* or Raphael's *Music to Disappear In*). Hit the Play button, turn the lights down low, lay down on your back, and close your eyes, listening to the piece (or pieces) of music that you have selected. Allow your mind to wander and begin to observe whatever images appear on the screen of your mind's eye. Note the colors, symbols, energies, and so on and merely observe where your mind takes you. Allow the music to help you paint a picture. As you do this, it's essential not to judge what you visualize, but rather

to simply observe and enjoy! Another option is to listen to a hemi-sync CD or audio track (The Monroe Institute), specially designed instrumental music that entrains the theta waves of each brain hemisphere for the ultimate music therapy experience (see www.hemi-Sync.com).

4. **The musical sounds of nature.** Nature provides an incredible soundtrack. In this exercise, you are invited to listen to the actual sounds of nature (e.g., a thunderstorm, waterfall, ocean surf, bird songs) or find an audio track with these recorded sounds. Give yourself about thirty minutes to listen to the natural sounds and simply allow your mind to wander wherever it will, without any judgment or reservations.

5. My top instrumental cuts of calming, relaxing music include the following:

a. _____

b. _____

c. _____

d. _____

e. _____

f. _____

g. _____

h. _____

i. _____

j. _____

k. _____

l. _____

m. _____

n. _____

o. _____

6. The top five energizing songs that lift my spirits are as follows:

a. _____

b. _____

c. _____

d. _____

e. _____

Massage Therapy

EXERCISE **23.1**

Self-Assessment: Bodywork

1. Have you ever had a session of massage therapy?   Yes   No
2. If so, what type(s) of bodywork did you have?

_____

3. Have you ever had a session of energy work?   Yes   No

     Reiki   Yes   No

     Healing touch   Yes   No

     Therapeutic touch   Yes   No

     Polarity therapy   Yes   No

     Reflexology   Yes   No

     Myofascial release   Yes   No

     Sports massage   Yes   No

     Craniosacral therapy   Yes   No

     Bio-energy healing   Yes   No

     Can you describe what one or more of these techniques felt like?

_____

_____

_____

_____

4. If you have not had a session of massage therapy, what is the primary reason (money, time, feelings of discomfort about the technique, not sure who to try)? Please explain.

_____

_____

5. Do you own a pet?   Yes   No

6. Have you experienced the benefits of pet therapy?   Yes   No

7. Have you experienced the benefits of aromatherapy?   Yes   No

    If so, what are some of your favorite aromatherapy scents?

_____

_____

_____

_____

Additional Thoughts on Massage Therapy, Pet Therapy, and Aromatherapy

_____

_____

_____

_____

_____

_____

_____

_____

_____

_____

_____

_____

_____

_____

_____

_____

EXERCISE **23.2**

Self-Massage

Ideally, the best massage you can receive is one that is performed by a licensed massage therapist who is both trained and experienced in many types of bodywork. Sadly, the muscles that produce the greatest amount of stress and tension are located on the back of your body—the hardest parts to reach! Fear not, however, because help is on the way, even if it's from your own set of hands. The following is a description of a few strategic areas that are prone to muscle tension and ways to relieve this with your own hands, beginning with the head, neck, and shoulders and continuing with the hands, legs, and feet.

Head

The temples, scalp, and eyes can be the target of significant muscle tension. Begin by taking your hands along the sides of each of your temples; with your fingertips, start to make small circles along the sides of your head above your eyes. After a series of five to ten circles moving in a clockwise direction, apply a bit more gentle pressure and reverse direction, going counterclockwise. Next, using your nondominant hand, extend your reach over the crown of your head and begin to knead the scalp in a clockwise direction, starting with gentle pressure on the right side of the head, then moving toward the back of the head, and finally working the left side of your head. Feel free to exchange hands, switching to the dominant hand. Then, place both hands over the crown of your head and, with your fingertips, massage the scalp with gentle pressure until you feel a slight tingling in your scalp. Be sure to take a slow, deep breath to promote good blood circulation. Relax your hand; then, reverse direction and repeat. When finished, close your eyes and take several comfortably slow, deep breaths.

Face

Your face repeatedly uses hundreds of muscles in the course of a day. A soft touch to these muscles always feels great. Begin by using the tips of your index and middle fingers of each hand to make small circles under and around each eye. Then progress by making small circles with the fingertips around the forehead, then around the cheek bones, and finally moving down the sides of the jaw and chin, continuing for several moments. Relax your hands by your sides and take three slow, deep breaths.

Neck

In the age of laptops and desktop computers, it is not uncommon to experience stiff necks, aching shoulders, and even headaches. As the midpoint between the head and shoulders, the neck deserves particular attention and muscular relief. Begin with both hands resting alongside the neck; then, leaning your head to the left, support your neck with your left hand and begin to knead the right side of your neck with your right hand. After several moments, lean your head to the right side and knead the left side of your neck with the opposite hand. Next, using the fingertips of each hand, gently make small circles along the sides of the neck. Then, taking your dominant hand, begin to knead the muscles of the back of neck, reaching from the base of the neck and slowly moving up toward the crown of the head, with the palm of your hand resting on the crown. Change hands when needed and repeat.

Shoulders

Continuing where the neck and shoulders meet, place your wrists alongside your neck, with your hands cupping the point where the neck and shoulder join. From here, begin a gentle kneading action at the center of your upper shoulders by applying gentle pressure along the sides of the spinal column. Then, with your nondominant hand, reach to the back of your dominant shoulder and continue the kneading action with your fingertips, again alongside the spinal column. Finally, work your way over to where the shoulder and arm connect by kneading the deltoid muscles. Relax your nondominant arm and take a few deep breaths. Then, using your dominant hand, repeat this process on the opposite side to your nondominant shoulder.

Hands

Your hands may not seem like the place to hold much tension, but given all the work they do—from typing at the computer keyboard to hundreds of other daily tasks—the hands also deserve significant attention. With your dominant hand, begin by making strong stroking motions from the base of the palm of your nondominant hand toward where the fingers connect to the hand. Then work your thumb and fingers along the sides of each of the fingers in your dominant hand. Finally, take the fingers of your dominant hand and stroke the back of your nondominant hand from the wrist to where the fingers attach. After several moments, release and relax both hands. Take a few comfortably slow, deep breaths, and then repeat this process using the opposite hand to massage your dominant hand.

Legs

Hold the left side of your left leg with your left hand. Then, using the palm of the right hand, apply gentle pressure with your thumb on the top of your left leg from the midthigh to the knee. Continue this stroking action along the inside of the upper leg as well for a few moments. Next, using both hands on the left leg, with your thumbs on the top (or sides) and the fingertips underneath, alternate kneading the hamstrings with first the right hand and then the left. Relax and take a few slow, deep breaths. Then, with one hand, reach for your calf muscle and knead it, squeezing and releasing the calf muscle between your thumb and fingertips. After several moments, release and relax your leg and take several slow, deep breaths. Repeat this technique with the opposite leg.

Feet

Considering all the work the feet do, from standing and walking to supporting your entire frame, both feet deserve much-needed comfort. Begin by placing your right foot on your left knee (or extending your reach to your right foot). Using both thumbs, begin to stroke the sole of the foot from the heel to the balls of the foot. After several moments take a slow, deep breath and repeat. With your fingertips, begin to work the area where the toes connect to the foot. Next, cup the heel of your foot with your left hand. With the fingers of your right hand, knead the tops of your feet, including the toes. Relax your foot back on the floor, rest your hands, and then repeat this procedure with the other foot.

Additional Thoughts: Please share your thoughts on the use of this exercise and perhaps how it compares to having a massage by a massage therapist.

_____

_____

_____

_____

_____

_____

_____

_____

_____

_____

_____

_____

_____

_____

_____

_____

_____

_____

T'ai Chi Ch'uan

EXERCISE **24.1**

The Yin and Yang of Life

T'ai Chi is based on the Taoist concept of seeking balance and going with the flow. The yin/yang symbol represents two opposite aspects coming together not in opposition but in union, creating the totality of the whole. The yin/yang symbol represents the balance of life.

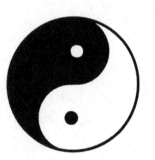

1. Take a moment to fill in the blanks of the following table.

Yin	Yang
_____	Heaven
Moon	_____
Autumn, winter	_____
_____	Masculine aspects
Cold, coolness	_____
_____	Brightness
Inside, interior	_____
_____	Things large and powerful
_____	The upper part

Yin	Yang
Water, rain	_____
_____	Movement
Night	_____
_____	The left side
The west and north	_____
_____	The back of the body
Exhaustion	_____
_____	Clarity
Development	_____
Conservation	_____
_____	Aggressiveness
Contraction	_____

2. Assuming you have either tried or regularly practice the art of T'ai Chi, please describe your impressions of this type of exercise as a means to promote relaxation.

_____

3. How do you see the effects (philosophy) of T'ai Chi carry over into other aspects of your life?

_____

_____

_____

4. The concept of balance is crucial to life, yet in this 24/7 society balance seems to be a rare commodity. List five things you can do to bring balance into your life.

a. _____

b. _____

c. _____

d. _____

e. _____

5. Please share any other comments you have regarding T'ai Chi here:

_____

_____

_____

_____

_____

_____

_____

_____

_____

_____

_____

_____

_____

_____

_____

_____

_____

_____

_____

_____

_____

_____

EXERCISE **24.2**

Energy: The Life Force

Look and it cannot be seen. Listen, and it cannot be heard.
Form that includes all forms. Subtle beyond all conception.
Lao Tzu, *Tao de Ching*

There is a life force of subtle energy that surrounds and permeates us all. The Chinese call this force *chi*. To harmonize with the universe, to move in unison with the energy, to move as free as running water, is to be at peace with or to be one with the universe. This harmony of energy promotes tranquility and inner peace.

To understand the concept of chi, it is helpful to view it from the cultural perspective in which it originated. Clinically speaking, the Chinese concept of health is quite different from that found in the Western hemisphere. Unlike those in the West who view health as the absence of disease and illness produced by bacteria and viruses, the Chinese view health as an unrestricted current of subtle energy that runs throughout the body. When chi, the subtle energy that flows through the body in a network of meridians, or "energy gates," is restricted or congested, the body is susceptible to physiological dysfunction. Hence, disturbances within the human energy field will result in physical symptoms of disease or illness.

According to Chinese medicine, it is not necessarily the bacterium or virus that causes physical dysfunction or disease; these are thought to be present everywhere. Rather, a state of poor health is thought to result from both internal and external factors, which ultimately do one in because of low resistance from nonharmonious (blocked) energy. Stated another way, these pathogens are constantly present; it is low resistance to them that makes one vulnerable to the disease. From a Chinese perspective, an unrestricted flow of energy helps maintain one's resistance to disturbing influences, be they biological, psychological, or sociological in nature.

Let's assume for a moment that the Chinese philosophy of health holds some merit—that a person's health status is based on the flow of energy. Perhaps you can gain a new perspective on your health from sensing your own energy levels. The following questions ask you to examine your energy level as the underlying current of your health status.

1. What do you notice about your level of energy and your health status? For example, are there times when your energy is low, only to be followed by catching a cold or flu? Describe what you feel like when you are energized and compare it with when you feel drained of energy.

2. Do certain circumstances, events, or episodes seem to drain your energy? What are they? Do you see patterns here?

3. When you are feeling run down, as if you are running on empty, what do you do to recharge yourself?

4. In Chinese culture, T'ai Chi, acupuncture, and acupressure are used to equilibrate the body's energy levels, clear the meridians, and restore one to a sense of well-being. Have you tried one or more of these techniques? If so, what are your impressions? If not, would you consider giving one of them a try?

Progressive Muscular Relaxation

EXERCISE **25.1**

Progressive Muscular Relaxation

Muscle tension is *the* number one symptom of stress. One often doesn't notice problems with tense muscles right away, but gradually muscle tension begins to distort the alignment of one's neck, shoulders, and spine. Muscle tension can affect the muscles of your jaw (known as temporomandibular joint dysfunction, or TMJD), the muscles of your shoulders, and perhaps most commonly the muscles of your lower back. Typically, it is the muscles on the back of the body that are most affected by neural tension and stress.

Progressive muscular relaxation (PMR) is one of the few relaxation techniques developed by a Western physician to respond to chronic stress associated with chronic pain. If you have never had muscle tension, consider yourself lucky. If you have had muscle tension of any type, consider yourself in good company. Even if you are somewhat relaxed, you can always become more relaxed, which is one benefit of PMR. (Reminder: PMR is not suggested for people who have been diagnosed with high blood pressure or hypertension.)

Assignment

Listen to the PMR exercise on the CD that accompanies *Managing Stress* and then answer the following.

1. What were your first impressions after completing the audio session of PMR? How did it make you feel? Did this exercise make you more aware of how slight muscle tension can be and still affect you?

_____

_____

_____

2. How did this technique compare with your experience with massage therapy, autogenic training, guided mental imagery, music therapy, or any other type of relaxation session you have had?

_____

_____

_____

3. Are you someone who suffers from chronic pain? How does a session of PMR affect the sensations of chronic pain (either directly in this muscle group or indirectly)?

_____

_____

_____

4. Make a list of four places in which you can do PMR in the course of a normal day to help you relieve muscle tension.

   a. _____

   b. _____

   c. _____

   d. _____

5. Please share any other comments regarding progressive muscular relaxation here:

_____

_____

_____

Chapter 26

Autogenic Training

EXERCISE **26.1**

Autogenic Training

Please listen to the autogenic training exercise on the CD that accompanies *Managing Stress* and then answer the following.

1. What were your first impressions when completing the audio session of autogenic training? How did it make you feel? Did this exercise make you more aware of how slight or even dramatic changes in perceptions of warmth and heaviness can make various body parts feel?

   _____

   _____

   _____

2. How did this technique compare with your experience with massage therapy, progressive muscular relaxation (PMR), guided mental imagery, music therapy, or any other type of relaxation session you have had?

   _____

   _____

   _____

3. Are you someone who suffers from chronic pain? How does a session of autogenic training affect the sensations of chronic pain (either directly in this muscle group or indirectly)?

   _____

   _____

   _____

265

4. Muscles are like sponges. When they are filled with blood, they are less tense (more pliable) than when there is little circulation. Dry muscles, like dry sponges, are very stiff. This technique is a great exercise to do before you fall asleep (insomniacs take note). If you have problems falling asleep at night, try this exercise and then write your impressions of how this worked.

_____

_____

_____

_____

5. Please share any other comments regarding autogenic training here:

_____

_____

_____

_____

_____

_____

_____

_____

_____

_____

_____

_____

_____

_____

_____

_____

_____

_____

EXERCISE **26.2**

The Power of Suggestion

Have you ever heard of neurolinguistic programming (NLP)? It is a behavior modification program designed by Richard Bandler and John Grinder based on the concept that words have specific meanings that our unconscious minds pick up on and use to direct our actions and, ultimately, even our state of health (Andreas and Falkner, 1994).

To understand this concept, it helps to know that our conscious mind makes up only a small portion (10 percent) of our total mind. This means that our unconscious mind is really both the navigator and pilot when it comes to behavior. Yet the conscious mind can override the system and cause some problems, especially when thoughts are not congruent with those of the unconscious mind. It gets complicated, but suffice it to say that although the unconscious mind thinks in terms of metaphors and similes, it takes quite literally that which the conscious mind articulates, even when the conscious mind speaks figuratively.

Neurolinguistic programming suggests that the power of words and expressions we use in everyday life can have a big impact on various aspects of our lives. For instance, to say "That sports car is to die for" may carry with it a foreshadowing of a date with the Grim Reaper. To say that your boss is a pain in the ass may, indeed, foreshadow some lower-back pain in the days or weeks to come.

To go one step further, the unconscious mind may suggest a host of expressions that may prophesize the direction of your health; for example, when you say something such as "My skin is so sensitive to sunlight that I am a walking tumor waiting to happen."

Neurolinguistic programming invites us to choose our words more cautiously and to get in the practice of thinking before we speak. Remember, the power of suggestion is quite tremendous, especially when the suggestion comes from the depths of your own mind.

1. Take notice of the selection of words you use in everyday conversation. Make note of expressions, idioms, colloquialisms, and vernacular that have both a literal and figurative meaning. List those that come to mind.

2. How often do you use negatives when you speak? If you are like most people, you probably use them quite often. It is said that the unconscious mind doesn't understand negatives. Try converting the negatives to positives. For example, when you say "I won't flunk this test," the unconscious mind translates this into "I will flunk this test." Jot down all of the negativisms you find yourself thinking or saying and then, next to each, write down a positive expression to use instead. For example, you could say "I will pass this test."

3. Take note of Freudian slips, that is, expressions that come out inadvertently when talking. Write these down as well and study them. By and large, they carry a message as well, if we take the time to listen.

Chapter 27

Biofeedback

Checking the Body's Pulses

If you have ever checked your pulse, taken your temperature, or watched yourself blush in the mirror, then you have done biofeedback. With the rapid advancement of high technology, the state of the art of biofeedback has changed dramatically since the first use of the lie detector test, which relied on galvanic skin response. By the time you read this workbook, advances in technology will probably have established sensors in clothing, computer mouses, and perhaps several more items that can regularly monitor various physiological parameters and tell you exactly how you are feeling at every moment. Welcome to the age of the biofeedback society.

Biofeedback, however, doesn't necessarily require expensive equipment or fancy high-tech gear. Some types of biofeedback can be done quite simply, such as monitoring your own breathing and checking your pulse before and after a relaxation session. This workbook assignment invites you to do just that.

Assignment

Count the number of breaths (breathing normally) you take in a one-minute period. If you are like most people, you will range between 14 and 16 breath cycles per minute. Next, check your resting heart rate. In a normal resting state it should be somewhere around 60 to 70 beats per minute.

Next, using one of the four tracks on the relaxation CD that accompanies *Managing Stress*, take yourself through this experience and then monitor both your respirations (breath cycles per minute) and resting heart rate (HR, in beats per minute) to determine how relaxed you became.

	Breath Cycle Before	*Breath Cycle After*
Track 1: Mountain Lake	_____	_____
Track 2: Progressive Muscular Relaxation	_____	_____
Track 3: Autogenics	_____	_____
Track 4: Rainbow Meditation	_____	_____

	Resting HR Before	*Resting HR After*
Track 1: Mountain Lake	_____	_____
Track 2: Progressive Muscular Relaxation	_____	_____
Track 3: Autogenics	_____	_____
Track 4: Rainbow Meditation	_____	_____

	General Sense of Well-Being Before	*General Sense of Well-Being After*
Track 1: Mountain Lake	_____	_____
Track 2: Progressive Muscular Relaxation	_____	_____
Track 3: Autogenics	_____	_____
Track 4: Rainbow Meditation	_____	_____

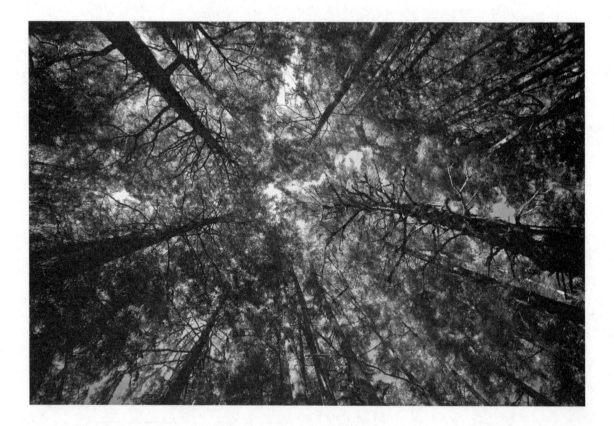

Physical Exercise, Nutrition, and Stress

EXERCISE 28.1

Physical Exercise

In simplest terms, we are physical animals with a human spirit. As human beings we were never meant to sit behind a desk for eight to ten hours a day. Human anatomy and physiology were designed to find a balance between motion and stillness, stress and homeostasis, exercise and relaxation. Some would say that the mounting incidence of disease and illness is a result of being out of physiological balance.

In this day and age, in which stress is at an all-time high, our bodies kick out several stress hormones, which, if not used for their intended purpose (to mobilize the body's systems for fight or flight), circulate throughout the body and tend to wreak havoc on various organs and constituents of the immune system. Physical exercise is considered the best way to keep the physiological systems of the body in balance, from stress hormones and adipose tissue to the integrity of bone cells and macrophages of the immune system.

Exercise doesn't have to be all that hard or time consuming. Perhaps more important than what you do is just making the time to do it. Mark Twain once said, "Oh, I get the urge to exercise every now and then, but I just lie down till it goes away." This may be humorous, but the truth of the matter is that physical exercise is what we need to promote the balance and integrity of our physiological systems. Although there is no doubt we seem to have a certain magnetic attraction to the couch and TV, this pattern of behavior has proved to be hazardous to our health.

1. Describe your exercise habits, including the formula for success (intensity, frequency, and duration of exercise).

2. What are your favorite activities? If for some reason you were injured and couldn't do your favorite activity, what would be your second option for exercise?

3. What do you do to motivate yourself when you are less than inspired to get up and out the door? What are some additional incentives to maintain a regular exercise regimen?

4. Most people say that they cannot find the time to exercise. Considering classes, studying, work, social obligations, and the like, it is hard to fit in everything. So

the question of priorities comes to mind. What are your priorities in terms of your health? Do you see your perspective changing in the course of your life? Right now, what can you do to find (make) the time to get physical exercise every day?

5. Sketch out a quick weekly program of exercise, including days to work out, time of day, and activity.

EXERCISE **28.2**

My Body, My Physique

Discovering your real self means the difference between freedom and the compulsions of conformity.
Maxwell Maltz

One often hears in California that "Nobody is ever satisfied with their hair." The same could be said about our bodies. We receive hundreds of messages a day from the media telling us that our physiques just aren't good enough. We spend hours and hours and gobs of money altering, complementing, adding, shifting, subtracting, and glamorizing various aspects of our bodies just to please other people in the hopes that we too can be pleased. Hair color, eye color, body weight (too much, too little), aerobic this, anaerobic that, add inches here, take off pounds there—it is fair to say that few people are completely satisfied with their bodies. But it doesn't have to be this way.

There is a strong connection between self-esteem and body image. The two go hand in hand. If your level of self-esteem is low, so too will be your body image. In his book *Psycho-Cybernetics*, Dr. Maxwell Maltz noted that many of his clients didn't seem all that much happier after receiving nose jobs and facelifts, which led him to the realization that the real change has to take place inside first.

So how do you feel about your body, your physique?

1. Describe your body. First list all the things you like about your body and explain why. Next, if so inclined, make a list of things you wish to improve.

2. Do you compare yourself with others? If you do, you're not alone. Actually, this is pretty common for both men and women, especially in college when your identity is still being formulated: Grooming yourself for that very important first impression can take priority over a term paper every time. So what is it you find yourself comparing with other people? Why?

3. The American public is obsessed with weight and weight gain. There is some good reason for this because of the relationship between obesity and diseases such as cancer, diabetes, and heart disease, but the concern has become an obsession for most people. Is your weight a concern for you? If so, how?

4. Taking to heart Maxwell Maltz's notion of making the first change within, can you think of any perceptions, attitudes, and beliefs you can begin to alter so that changes you do make to your physique are long-lasting ones with which you feel content?

_____

_____

_____

_____

_____

273

EXERCISE **28.3**

My Circadian Rhythms

Your body runs on a 24-hour-plus clock, based on the earth spinning on its axis around the sun. Research shows that people who keep to a regular schedule tend to be healthier (fewer colds, flus, etc.) than those whose lifestyle behaviors tend to be more erratic, because these tend to stress the body. In this exercise you are asked to monitor your lifestyle behaviors based on the time of day that these occur for the period of a full week.

Week of _____

Circadian Rhythms	Sun.	Mon.	Tue.	Wed.	Thurs.	Fri.	Sat.
1. Time that you awake each morning							
2. Time that you go to bed							
3. Time that you fall asleep							
4. Time that you eat breakfast							
5. Time that you eat lunch							
6. Time that you eat dinner							
7. Times that you snack							
8. Times of bowel movements							
9. Times that you exercise							
10. Times that you have sex							
11. Other regular activities							

EXERCISE **28.4**

My Body's Rhythms

The body has an internal clock that runs on a 24- to 25-hour day. If you were to lock yourself away from all the natural elements (sunlight, temperature fluctuations, etc.) and the grip of technology (TVs, radios, computers, etc.), as some people have for research purposes, your body would fall into a natural pattern, its *circadian rhythm*. To a large extent, these rhythms are based on and are strongly influenced by the elements of the natural world: the earth's rotation, the gravitational pull, the earth's axis, and several other influences of which we are probably not even aware.

Other rhythms influence our bodies as well: *infradian rhythms* (less than 24-hour cycles) such as stomach contractions for hunger and rapid eye movement cycles, and *ultradian rhythms* (more than 24-hour cycles), such as menstrual periods and red blood cell formation.

As we continue to embrace the achievements of high technology and separate ourselves even further from the reach of nature, we throw off our body's natural rhythms. When these rhythms are thrown off for too long a time, various organs that depend on the regularity of these rhythms go into a state of dysfunction.

College life holds no particular order for body rhythms. You can eat dinner one day at 6:00 P.M. and the next day at 9:30 P.M. We won't even talk about sleep! Perhaps at a young age your body can rebound from these cyclical irregularities. More likely than not, though, regular disruptions in the body's rhythms will manifest quickly in various ways such as irritability, fatigue, lack of hunger, restless sleep and insomnia, low resistance to illness, and lowered mental capacities.

1. What is your general sense of your body's rhythms?

2. Do you keep to a regular schedule with regard to eating, sleeping, and exercise? Or does the time you do these vary from day to day?

3. How closely are you connected with nature? Do you spend time outdoors every day? Do you find yourself more tired, perhaps even more irritable, as we shift from autumn into winter? Do you find yourself more energized, perhaps more positive or optimistic, as we shift from winter to spring?

4. If you are a woman, what is the regularity of your menstrual period? Can you identify a pattern with your nutritional habits, stress levels, and other daily rituals that may influence your menses?

_____

_____

_____

_____

_____

*48
18 /
66*

EXERCISE **28.5**

Stress-Related Eating Behaviors

Please read the following statements and circle the appropriate answer. Then tally the total to determine your score using the key below.

48   16

4 = Always	3 = Often	2 = Sometimes	1 = Rarely	0 = Never

1. I tend to skip breakfast on a regular basis.	④	3	2	1	0
2. On average, two or three meals are prepared outside the home each day.	④	3	2	1	0
3. I drink more than one cup of coffee or tea a day.	④	3	2	1	0
4. I tend to drink more than one soda/pop per day.	④	3	2	1	0
5. I commonly snack between meals.	④	3	2	1	0
6. When in a hurry, I usually eat at fast food places.	④	3	2	1	0
7. I tend to snack while watching television.	4	③	2	1	0
8. I tend to put salt on my food before tasting it.	4	3	2	1	⓪
9. I drink fewer than eight glasses of water a day.	④	3	2	1	0
10. I tend to satisfy my sweet tooth daily.	④	3	2	1	0
11. When preparing meals at home, I usually don't cook from scratch.	4	③	2	1	0
12. Honestly, my eating habits lean toward fast, junk, processed foods.	④	3	2	1	0
13. I eat fewer than four to five servings of fresh vegetables per day.	④	3	2	1	0
14. I drink at least one glass of wine, beer, or alcohol a day.	④	3	2	1	0
15. My meals are eaten sporadically throughout the day rather than at regularly scheduled times.	4	③	2	1	0
16. I don't usually cook with fresh herbs and spices.	4	③	2	1	0
17. I usually don't make a habit of eating organic fruits and veggies.	④	3	2	1	0
18. My biggest meal of the day is usually eaten after 7:00 P.M.	4	③	2	1	0
19. For the most part, my vitamins and minerals come from the foods I eat.	4	3	2	1	⓪
20. Artificial sweeteners are in many of the foods I eat.	4	③	2	1	0

Total score   *66*

Scoring Key

A score of more than 20 points indicates that your eating behaviors are not conducive to reducing stress. A score of more than 30 suggests that your eating habits may seriously compromise the integrity of your immune system.

EXERCISE **28.6**

Self-Assessment: Nutritional Eating Habits

1. Do you regularly consume caffeine?   Yes   No

2. List the foods that you ingest that contain caffeine (e.g., coffee, tea, sodas, chocolate) and the estimated amounts you consume per day.

   Type of Food with Caffeine   *Amount per Day*

   a. _____   _____

   b. _____   _____

   c. _____   _____

   d. _____   _____

   e. _____   _____

   f. _____   _____

3. Do you take vitamin supplements?   Yes   No

   If yes, what kinds?

   _____

4. Do you frequently use table salt?   Yes   No

5. Do you eat one or more meals that are prepared outside the home daily?   Yes   No

6. Do you consume junk food (from vending machines or convenience stores) regularly?   Yes   No

7. Do you eat cereals that contain sugar?   Yes   No

8. Do you drink a lot of soft drinks?   Yes   No

9. Do you find that when you are stressed you tend to eat more?   Yes   No

10. Do you find that when you are angry you tend to eat more?   Yes   No

11. Do you eat a wide variety of fruits and vegetables?   Yes   No

12. Do you eat foods (e.g., fish and nuts) with the essentials oils (omega-3 and omega-6)?   Yes   No

13. Do you tend to eat quickly (e.g., to wolf down your food)?   Yes   No

14. Do you tend to drink alcohol as a means to relax?   Yes   No

15. List your top five comfort foods:

    a. _____

    b. _____

    c. _____

    d. _____

    e. _____

16. Describe any other eating habits that you associate with a stressed lifestyle:

    _____

    _____

    _____

    _____

    _____

    _____

    _____

    _____

    _____

    _____

    _____

    _____

    _____

    _____

    _____

    _____

    _____

    _____

    _____

    _____

    _____

    _____

EXERCISE **28.7**

The Rainbow Diet

Food color is more important than just having a nice presentation on your dinner plate. Each color holds a specific vibration in the spectrum of light. When this is combined with the nutrient value of food, it can help to enhance the health of the physical body. In the science of subtle energies, each of the body's primary chakras is associated with a specific color (see accompanying chart). It is thought that eating fruits and vegetables associated with the color of various chakras provides healthy energy to that specific region. For example, women with urinary tract infections (root chakra) are encouraged to drink cranberry juice (red). Diabetic people with macular problems are encouraged to eat blueberries and take the herb bilberry (blue). Moreover, recent research suggests that the active ingredients in fruits and vegetables that give them their color, called bioflavonoids, help prevent cancer. Regardless of Eastern philosophies or Western science, the bottom line is to eat a good variety of fruits and vegetables.

The following table identifies the seven chakras, their respective body regions, and the color associated with each chakra or region. List five fruits, veggies, or herbs for each color.

Chakra	Body Region	Color	Food Choices
7: Crown	Pineal	Purple	_____
6: Brow	Pituitary	Indigo	_____
5: Throat	Thymus	Aqua blue	_____
4: Heart	Heart	Green	_____
3: Solar plexus	Adrenals	Yellow	_____
2: Navel	Spleen	Orange	_____
1: Root	Gonads	Red	_____

Additional Thoughts:

_____

_____

_____

_____

_____

_____

EXERCISE **28.8**

Food, Glorious Food!

If there is one aspect of health and wellness that maintains an air of controversy, it is the topic of nutrition. It seems that a day doesn't go by on which some new scientific study contradicts the findings of a previous study published months earlier. This is good for you, that is bad for you, this causes cancer, that promotes the immune system, and so on. In the search for truth, most people just shrug their shoulders, toss up their arms, and give up.

This we do know: The American diet is top-heavy in saturated fats, sugars, salts, and cholesterol. More Americans eat meals prepared outside the home than meals cooked at home. These meals are prepared with lots of fats, and hydrogenated oils contain trans fatty acids that wreak havoc on the integrity of each cell, setting the stage for cancer and heart disease. Fiber content in American diets is extremely low, and this too is thought to be a risk factor for cancer, particularly colon cancer. Let's face it, for a society on the go, the American diet is stopping us dead in our tracks.

You may have heard that the college years are the formative years. This is the chance to explore your freedoms without parental censorship. In terms of food, this means you can eat whatever you want, whenever you want; you don't have to answer to anyone, except yourself. Everyone knows that college students love food but, as a rule, hate to cook, even if there were time to do so. These factors can set the stage for some pretty unhealthy nutritional habits, which can last a lifetime if they go unaltered.

So let's talk eating habits!

1. Describe your eating habits: How many meals do you eat a day? What is your typical day like? How many meals do you eat outside the home each day? Do you cook meals from scratch, or are you the kind of person who buys a lot of precooked meals?

2. Eating out is like a reward: Someone else does the cooking, someone else serves the food to you, and, thank God, someone else cleans the dishes. Notwithstanding the motto "Some is good, more is better," eating out can be as much a hazard to your physical health as it is a reward to your mental health. When you do go out to eat, what types of food selections do you make? Are they pretty much the same over time? Do you ask for no MSG when you order Chinese food? Limit diet sodas to just one? Opt for salad without dressing? Do you avoid deep-fried foods (onion rings, french fries, cheese sticks)? These are just some of the things to be aware of when making healthy eating choices.

3. Do you take vitamin and mineral supplements? If you eat a well-balanced diet, it is probably not necessary. Conventional wisdom, however, suggests that in this day and age no one eats enough well-balanced meals to get what they need in terms of vitamins and minerals. If you do take supplements, are they synthesized or lyophilized? Since the body cannot metabolize synthesized supplements very well, you may be wasting your money. Please describe your habits here.

_____

_____

_____

_____

_____

_____

_____

_____

_____

_____

_____

_____

_____

_____

_____

_____

_____

_____

_____

_____

_____

_____

_____

_____

_____

_____

_____

EXERCISE **28.9**

Fast Food Nation

*Nobody in America is forced to buy fast food. The first step
toward meaningful change is far the easiest: stop buying it!*
Eric Schlosser, *Fast Food Nation*

In 2001 Eric Schlosser wrote a landmark book entitled *Fast Food Nation*, in which he explored behind the scenes of the fast food industry. In 2006 this book was made into a Hollywood movie. What began as an article for *Rolling Stone* evolved into a year-long investigation for his book. What he reveals about the fast food industry (mostly McDonald's, since that company epitomizes it) is enough to make your stomach turn.

Here are some interesting facts from his book:

- In 1970, Americans spent about $6 billion on fast food; in 2010, they spent more than $120 billion.
- Americans now spend more money on fast food than on higher education.
- On any given day about 25 percent of the adult population visits a fast food restaurant.
- McDonald's has employed an estimated one of every eight workers in the United States.
- Billions are spent each year to market fast food to toddlers to build life-long brand-name loyalty.
- Schools that once housed cafeterias now only carry fast food restaurants.
- Only Santa Claus has higher face recognition than Ronald McDonald among fictional characters.
- What we eat (processed foods) has changed more in the last 40 years than in the previous 4,000.
- The United States has more prison inmates than full-time farmers.
- Every day approximately 200,000 people are sickened by a foodborne disease. The most common cause of foodborne outbreaks has been the consumption of undercooked ground beef containing *E. coli* O157:H7 (from animal feces).
- A single animal infected with *E. coli* O157:H7 can contaminate 32,000 pounds of that ground beef.
- A single fast food hamburger now contains meat from dozens or even hundreds of different cattle.

More than likely you are among the millions of people who participate in the daily fast food ritual. Reasons given by most college students include cost and convenience. It certainly isn't nutrients.

This journal theme asks you to explore your fast food and junk food habits: What are they, and why do you feel you have these habits? Sometimes, by actually taking time to write down what we do in terms of our behaviors, we begin to see patterns that we don't normally see day to day. Finally, contemplate this thought. Schlosser suggests that the fast food industry has had a tremendous impact on American society as a whole, from poor-quality service to disposable meals. Please share your comments on this aspect as well.

_____

_____

_____

_____

_____

_____

_____

_____

_____

_____

_____

_____

_____

_____

_____

_____

_____

_____

EXERCISE **28.10**

Frankenfoods: The Monster Called GMOs

Let food be your medicine and medicine be your food.
Hippocrates, father of Western medicine

What is your relationship with food? Do you buy your food frozen, prepackaged, freeze-dried, or canned? Do you cook your own food or does someone typically do it for you? It is interesting to note that Americans are up in arms about human cloning, yet no one seems to even notice that scientists are splicing the DNA of flounder into tomatoes, the genes of rats into hogs, and the pesticide Roundup into the DNA of corn. The Kellogg Company had to recall millions of boxes of Corn Flakes in 2000, and Taco Bell recalled thousands of taco shells because of the hazards of genetically modified foods. Those people who are allergic to peanuts now have to watch the corn products they eat. Cross-species gene splicing has made corn a dangerous food to consume. In fact, many food allergies are thought to be related to genetically modified organisms (GMOs).

Food experts suggest that as many as 70 percent of the produce and processed foods in the grocery store are genetically modified. At the top of the list are tomatoes (a category that includes ketchup, tomato sauce, and salsa), corn, and soy. By the time you read this there could be many, many more. Effective lobbying efforts in Congress by the Monsanto Corporation have allowed these foods to go unlabeled.

1. What types of foods do you buy in the grocery store?
2. What percentage of meals do you eat outside the home each week?
3. What percentage of foods do you buy that are organic?
4. Are you allergic to any foods? If so, which ones? Have you noticed being allergic to more foods in the past five years than before this time when GMOs were introduced?
5. Go online to your favorite search engine and type in the words *Frankenfoods* or *GMO*. Check out three or four websites and write down some of the highlights you find.
6. After you have done this, take a few minutes to write down your thoughts on the topic of Frankenfoods.

_____

_____

_____

_____

_____

_____

EXERCISE **28.11**

Is Fat Really Where It's At?

Transfatty acids are so unnatural, even bacteria won't go near them!
Doug Margel, D.O.

Perhaps you have heard—America has a weight problem. Over 50 percent of Americans are considered obese by several standards, including body composition tests and body mass index (BMI). Although several factors are related to obesity, one of the first factors to address is the types of foods that we eat. Much attention has been placed on saturated fat and cholesterol, but this is only the tip of the iceberg, if not the ever-evolving food guide pyramid.

In the early twentieth century, scientists began to experiment with lipids to reduce the rate of rancidity (e.g., Crisco oil). In essence, they were looking for ways to prolong the shelf life of processed foods that contained fat. Their legacy has haunted us ever since. It is virtually impossible to find any packaged food without "partially hydrogenated oil" listed in the ingredients. Examples include everything from cookies and potato chips to cereal, pancake mix, and peanut butter. Hydrogenation of oils (making a lipid a saturated fat at room temperature) created trans fatty acids. Current research suggests that these act like free radicals. In essence, they destroy the integrity of various cells, including the cell wall, DNA, RNA, and mitochondria. Transfatty acids are linked to both coronary heart disease and cancer. They are also most definitely linked to the obesity problem in America. Why? Because these types of fats are not natural, and once absorbed into the body, the body has no idea what to do with them. In small amounts they may not appear to do much, but over time they can cause a real problem. Here is some alarming news: Despite the fact that food companies are required to place trans fats on food labels, because of the way the laws were written, several foods that are labeled "No trans fats" still contain partially hydrogenated oils (read the labels).

Here is your assignment: Go into your kitchen and open the cupboards and refrigerator. Start looking at the list of ingredients of the foods you find and make a list. Most likely you will be amazed at what you find.

Here is another problem: Your body has to have omega-3s (codfish oils and flaxseed oil) and omega-6s (vegetable oils). But nowhere on the food guide pyramid does it say you have to have these. These are called essential fatty acids because your body cannot make them—they have to be consumed from the foods you eat. The problem is that in our fat-phobic society, people are not getting the correct balance of essential fatty acids (not enough omega-3s and too much of omega-6s). A lack of essential fatty acids is now thought to be a determining factor in several chronic diseases. Are you getting enough of these? Are you getting the right balance? Go back into the kitchen and see whether these sources of oil are in your fridge. Come back and report what you find.

EXERCISE **28.12**

The Serotonin Blues

It's hard to believe that in a country as great as the United States, where the living standard is the envy of almost every other nation in the world, about one-third of the population is diagnosed with or being medically treated for depression. Something is terribly wrong with this picture. Although the American dream states that "You can have it all," this promise certainly has its drawbacks. (For one thing, where would you put it?)

Medical scientists have known for several decades that at the biochemical level, depression is related to a decrease in the hormone serotonin, a special neurotransmitter that regulates a great many physiological processes in the body. The relationship between and among neurotransmitters in the brain is complex, to say the least. Serotonin works in conjunction with dopamine and melatonin as well as several other neuropeptides. These in turn also seem to have a great effect on our emotions.

The biomedical model of well-being is myopic. It only sees brain chemistry having an effect on emotions, not the other way around. The biochemical model also falls short of recognizing that many of the foods we eat play a significant role in brain neurochemistry. These include a host of artificial flavors, colors, preservatives, and sweeteners.

Freud once said that depression is anger turned inward. Indeed, depression is more complex than the levels of serotonin produced in the brain. But this is a good place to start to look and see how we might be affected.

Most likely there is a good chance that you or someone you know has been depressed. This journal theme is dedicated to the topic of depression. It offers you a chance to write about how you feel when you become emotionally overwhelmed. Thinking holistically, what steps can you take to move out of the shadow of depression through mind, body, spirit, and emotions?

_____

_____

_____

_____

_____

_____

_____

_____

EXERCISE **28.13**

Mandala for Personal Health: Your Holistic Stress-Management Strategy

This mandala exercise invites you to use this symbol of wholeness as both a reminder of your true self and a compass to help get you there, should you lose your way in the course of daily events and circumstances that tend to cloud your vision and perspective. Using the mandala below, first write your name in the center. Next, keeping in mind that many activities cross the lines between these quadrants, write in each respective quadrant your ideas, skills and techniques, exercises, and habits that allow you to achieve inner peace through the integration, balance, and harmony of mind, body, spirit, and emotions. For example, let's take the quadrant for physical well-being. You might consider writing down ideas for your personal exercise program, new or improved eating habits, sleep habits, and perhaps even acupuncture and a massage. List those things that you either currently do or wish to include in your life routine. When you finish, place the mandala where you can see it regularly to serve as a reminder to guide you to your optimal health potential. You may also consider doing a larger version by cutting out color photographs and words from magazines to bring this mandala to a whole new level.

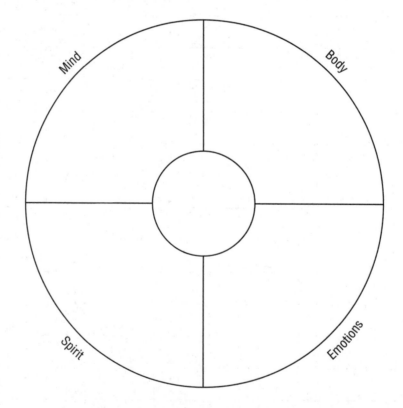

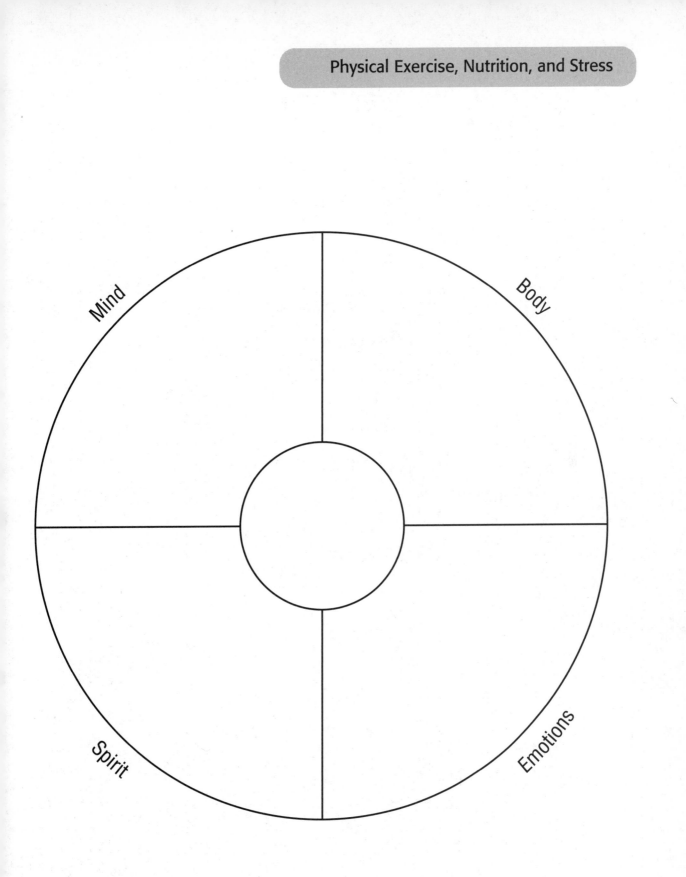

Effective
Relaxation Techniques

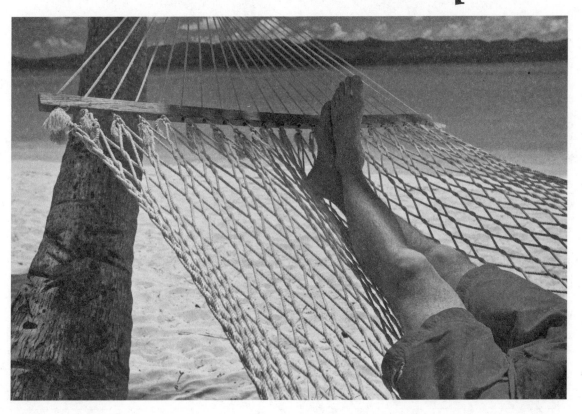

EXERCISE **IV.A**

The Art of Calm: Relaxation through the Five Senses

Please list ten ideas for relaxation for each of the five senses. Note that a sixth category, the divine sense, was added for any ideas that might be a combination of these or perhaps something beyond the five senses (e.g., watching a child being born). Describe each in a few words to a sentence. Be as specific as possible, and be creative!

The Sense of Sight

1. _____
2. _____
3. _____
4. _____
5. _____
6. _____
7. _____
8. _____
9. _____
10. _____

The Sense of Taste

1. _____
2. _____
3. _____
4. _____
5. _____
6. _____
7. _____
8. _____
9. _____
10. _____

The Sense of Sound

1. _____
2. _____
3. _____
4. _____
5. _____
6. _____
7. _____

The Sense of Touch

1. _____
2. _____
3. _____
4. _____
5. _____
6. _____
7. _____

8. _____

9. _____

10. _____

8. _____

9. _____

10. _____

The Sense of Smell

1. _____

2. _____

3. _____

4. _____

5. _____

6. _____

7. _____

8. _____

9. _____

10. _____

The Divine Sense

1. _____

2. _____

3. _____

4. _____

5. _____

6. _____

7. _____

8. _____

9. _____

10. _____

EXERCISE **IV.B**

Relaxation Survival Kit

A *relaxation survival kit* is like your personal first-aid kit for stress. Keep it well stocked with things that nurture or sustain your personal sense of homeostasis—in this case, homeostasis that comes from pleasing one or all of the five senses. Just like a first-aid kit, be sure to replace any items that have been used—such as chocolate (taste)—so that in the event of another personal disaster or day from hell, you can pull out your kit and put yourself back on the path toward inner peace. To start this process, begin by making a list of the items you wish to include in your relaxation kit, and then use this list as a means of keeping inventory.

Sight

1. _____

2. _____

Sound

1. _____

2. _____

Taste

1. _____

2. _____

Touch

1. _____

2. _____

Smell

1. _____

2. _____

Additional Items

1. _____

2. _____